Diffuse Large B-Cell Lymphoma

About the NCCN Guidelines for Patients®

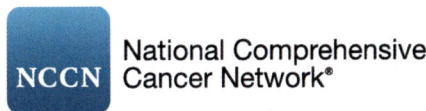 National Comprehensive Cancer Network®

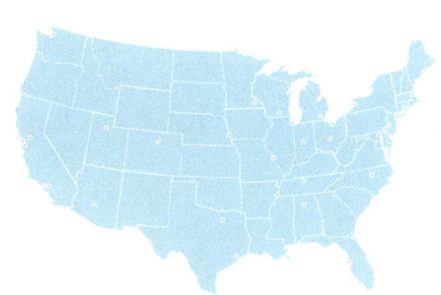

Did you know that top cancer centers across the United States work together to improve cancer care? This alliance of leading cancer centers is called the National Comprehensive Cancer Network® (NCCN®).

Cancer care is always changing. NCCN develops evidence-based cancer care recommendations used by health care providers worldwide. These frequently updated recommendations are the NCCN Clinical Practice Guidelines in Oncology (NCCN Guidelines®). The NCCN Guidelines for Patients plainly explain these expert recommendations for people with cancer and caregivers.

These NCCN Guidelines for Patients are based on the NCCN Clinical Practice Guidelines in Oncology (NCCN Guidelines®) for B-Cell Lymphomas Version 2.2025 – February 10, 2025

View the NCCN Guidelines for Patients free online	Find an NCCN Cancer Center near you
NCCN.org/patientguidelines	NCCN.org/cancercenters

Connect with us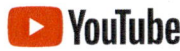

Diffuse Large B-Cell Lymphomas

Supporters

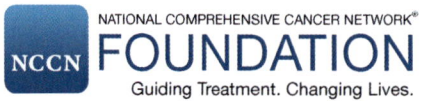

NCCN Guidelines for Patients are supported by funding from the NCCN Foundation®

NCCN Foundation gratefully acknowledges the following corporate supporters for helping to make available these NCCN Guidelines for Patients: AstraZeneca; Genmab US, Inc.; Incyte Corporation; Kite, a Gilead Company; and Pfizer Inc.

NCCN independently adapts, updates, and hosts the NCCN Guidelines for Patients. Our corporate supporters do not participate in the development of the NCCN Guidelines for Patients and are not responsible for the content and recommendations contained therein.

To make a gift or learn more, visit online or email

NCCNFoundation.org/donate

PatientGuidelines@NCCN.org

Contents

4   About DLBCL

9   Testing for DLBCL

25   Types of treatment

36   Supportive care

42   Stages 1, 2, 3, and 4

49   Relapsed and refractory disease

56   ALK-positive large B-cell lymphomas

59   Primary mediastinal large B-cell lymphomas

64   High-grade B-cell lymphomas

68   Mediastinal gray zone lymphomas

72   Primary cutaneous DLBCL, leg type

77   Other resources

81   Words to know

84   NCCN Contributors

85   NCCN Cancer Centers

88   Index

© 2025 National Comprehensive Cancer Network, Inc. All rights reserved. NCCN Guidelines for Patients and illustrations herein may not be reproduced in any form for any purpose without the express written permission of NCCN. No one, including doctors or patients, may use the NCCN Guidelines for Patients for any commercial purpose and may not claim, represent, or imply that the NCCN Guidelines for Patients that have been modified in any manner are derived from, based on, related to, or arise out of the NCCN Guidelines for Patients. The NCCN Guidelines are a work in progress that may be redefined as often as new significant data become available. NCCN makes no warranties of any kind whatsoever regarding its content, use, or application and disclaims any responsibility for its application or use in any way.

NCCN Foundation seeks to support the millions of patients and their families affected by a cancer diagnosis by funding and distributing NCCN Guidelines for Patients. NCCN Foundation is also committed to advancing cancer treatment by funding the nation's promising doctors at the center of innovation in cancer research. For more details and the full library of patient and caregiver resources, visit NCCN.org/patients.

National Comprehensive Cancer Network (NCCN) and NCCN Foundation
3025 Chemical Road, Suite 100, Plymouth Meeting, PA 19462 USA

1
About DLBCL

5 What is DLBCL?

5 What are lymphocytes?

6 What is the lymphatic system?

7 What's in this book?

8 What can you do to get the best care?

1 About DLBCL » What is DLBCL? » What are lymphocytes?

Diffuse large B-cell lymphoma (DLBCL) develops from lymphocytes, a type of white blood cell. It is a fast-growing cancer, affecting tissues and organs such as bone marrow, spleen, thymus, lymph nodes, lymphatic vessels, and other parts of the body.

What is DLBCL?

Diffuse large B-cell lymphoma (DLBCL) is the most common type of non-Hodgkin lymphoma (NHL). NHLs develop from lymphocytes, a type of white blood cell. In DLBCL, B-cell lymphocytes grow out of control and form tumors. Tumors are commonly found in lymph nodes, spleen, liver, bone marrow, or other tissues and organs. DLBCL can cause swollen lymph nodes. Symptoms can include fever, night sweats, fatigue, and weight loss. These symptoms are referred to as B symptoms. Not everyone has the same symptoms and tumors can be found anywhere in the body.

What are lymphocytes?

White blood cells (WBCs or leukocytes) include granulocytes, monocytes, and lymphocytes. A lymphocyte is a type of white blood cell that helps fight and prevent infection. Lymphocytes are found in blood and lymph tissue, and every organ in the body. Lymph tissue includes lymph vessels and lymph nodes. Lymphocytes normally grow in response to infection or inflammation. When they grow on their own without proper regulation, they can develop into lymphoma.

There are 3 main types of lymphocytes:

- **B lymphocytes or B cells** make antibodies. An antibody is a protein that specifically targets infections or cancer cells and recruits other parts of the immune system.
- **T lymphocytes or T cells** help fight infections, kill tumor cells, and control immune responses.
- **Natural killer (NK) cells** can kill tumor cells or virus-infected cells.

DLBCL arises from B cells. B cells mature into plasma cells, which produce antibodies that are used to attack invading bacteria, viruses, and toxins. The antibody molecules latch onto and destroy invading viruses or bacteria by recruiting other components of the immune system. Cancers of plasma cells are multiple myeloma and not lymphoma.

What is the lymphatic system?

DLBCL affects the lymphatic system. The lymphatic or lymph system is a major part of the body's immune system. It is a germ-fighting network of tissues and organs that includes the bone marrow, spleen, thymus, lymph nodes, and lymphatic vessels.

Lymphatic vessels are a network of thin tubes that carry lymphatic fluid (lymph) and white blood cells into all the tissues of the body. Lymph gives cells water and food. White blood cells, such as lymphocytes, help fight infection and disease.

As lymph travels throughout your body, it passes through hundreds of small bean-shaped structures called lymph nodes. Lymph nodes make immune cells that help the body fight infection. They also filter the lymph fluid and remove foreign material such as bacteria and cancer cells.

Lymph nodes can swell due to infections, inflammation, or cancers. Many types of lymphoma, including DLBCL, cause painless enlargement of lymph nodes as a result of cancer cell growth.

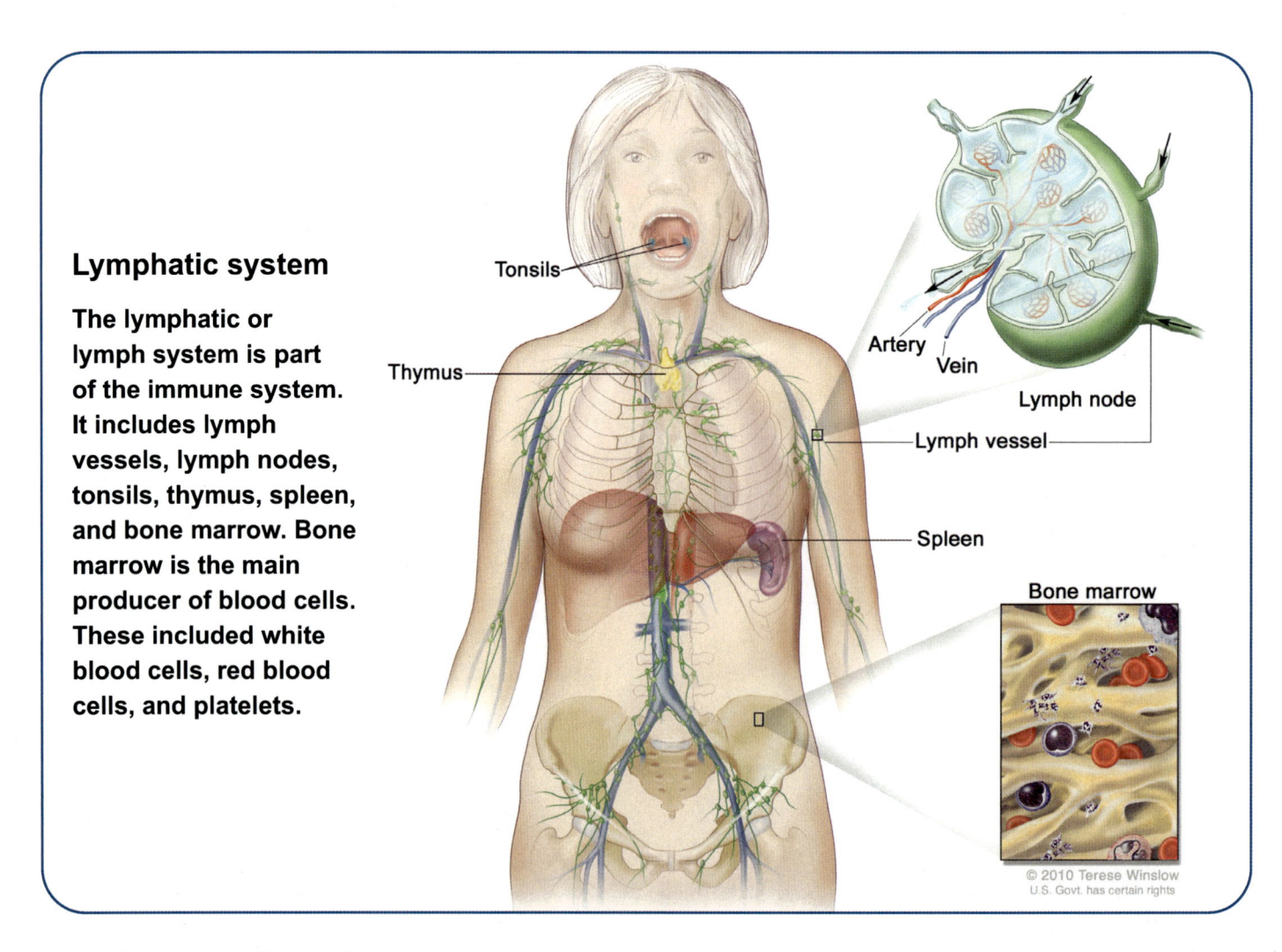

Lymphatic system

The lymphatic or lymph system is part of the immune system. It includes lymph vessels, lymph nodes, tonsils, thymus, spleen, and bone marrow. Bone marrow is the main producer of blood cells. These included white blood cells, red blood cells, and platelets.

1 About DLBCL » What's in this book?

What's in this book?

This book is organized into the following chapters:

Chapter 2: Testing for DLBCL provides an overview of tests you might receive, and the role of genetic and biomarker mutation testing.

Chapter 3: Types of treatment gives a general overview of DLBCL treatment.

Chapter 4: Supportive care gives an overview of what supportive care is and possible side effects of treatment.

Chapter 5: Stages 1, 2, 3, and 4 discusses treatment of DLBCL based on cancer stage.

Chapter 6: Relapsed and refractory disease discuss treatment for DLBCL that has returned or progressed during treatment.

Chapter 7: ALK-positive large B-cell lymphomas discusses treatment of large B-cell lymphomas with a mutation in the anaplastic lymphoma kinase (ALK) gene.

Chapter 8: Primary mediastinal large B-cell lymphomas discusses treatment of large B-cell lymphoma that develops in the area behind the breastbone called the mediastinum.

Chapter 9: High-grade B-cell lymphomas discusses treatment for very aggressive, fast-dividing tumors such as those with high-risk features or certain mutations and gene rearrangements (*MYC* with *BCL2* or *MYC* with *BCL6*).

Chapter 10: Mediastinal gray zone lymphomas have overlapping features of primary mediastinal B-cell lymphoma (PMBL) and Hodgkin lymphoma (HL). This chapter discusses treatment of mediastinal gray zone lymphomas (MGZL).

Chapter 11: Primary cutaneous DLBCL, leg type discusses treatment for a type of DLBCL that causes skin lesions.

Chapter 12: Other resources provide information on patient advocacy groups and where to get help.

Why you should read this book

Making decisions about cancer care can be stressful. You may need to make tough decisions under pressure about complex choices.

The NCCN Guidelines for Patients are trusted by patients and providers. They clearly explain current care recommendations made by respected experts in the field. Recommendations are based on the latest research and practices at leading cancer centers.

Cancer care is not the same for everyone. By following expert recommendations for your situation, you are more likely to improve your care and have better outcomes as a result. Use this book as your guide to find the information you need to make important decisions.

1 About DLBCL » What can you do to get the best care?

What can you do to get the best care?

Advocate for yourself. You have an important role to play in your care. In fact, you're more likely to get the care you want by asking questions and making shared decisions with your care team. Consider seeking the opinion of a DLBCL specialist.

The NCCN Guidelines for Patients will help you understand cancer care. With better understanding, you'll be more prepared to discuss your care with your team and share your concerns. Many people feel more satisfied when they play an active role in their care.

You may not know what to ask your care team. That's common. Each chapter in this book ends with an important section called Questions to ask. These suggested questions will help you get more information on all aspects of your care.

Take the next step and keep reading to learn what is the best care for you!

We want your feedback!

Our goal is to provide helpful and easy-to-understand information on cancer. Take our survey to let us know what we got right and what we could do better.
NCCN.org/patients/feedback

2
Testing for DLBCL

10 Types of large B-cell lymphomas

11 General health tests

12 Fertility (all genders)

13 Blood tests

15 Biopsy

16 Immunophenotyping

18 Testing for DLBCL biomarker and genetic changes

21 Imaging tests

23 Lumbar puncture

23 Heart tests

24 Key points

24 Questions to ask

2 Testing for DLBCL » Types of large B-cell lymphomas

Accurate testing is needed to diagnose and treat diffuse large B-cell lymphoma (DLBCL). This chapter presents an overview of possible tests you might receive and what to expect.

Types of large B-cell lymphomas

Large B-cell lymphomas (LBCLs) are characterized by large, abnormal B-cells, a type of white blood cell. There are many types of large B-cell lymphomas. Diffuse large B-cell lymphoma (DLBCL) is just one type. Accurate testing is needed to determine the type of LBCL. For types of LBCL, **see Guide 1.**

Guide 1
Large B-cell lymphoma (LBCL) types

Diffuse large B-cell lymphoma (DLBCL)	Intravascular LBCL
DLBCL, not otherwise specified (DLBCL-NOS)	DLBCL associated with chronic inflammation
ALK-positive large B-cell lymphoma (LBCL)	Fibrin-associated DLBCL
Mediastinal gray zone lymphoma (MGZL)	EBV-positive DLBCL, NOS
Primary mediastinal large B-cell lymphoma (PMBL)	T-cell/histiocyte-rich LBCL
Primary cutaneous DLBCL, leg type (PC-DLBCL, leg type)	LBCL with *IRF4/MUM1* rearrangement
High-grade B-cell lymphoma (HGBL)	LBCL with 11q aberration/HGBL with 11q aberrations
High-grade B-cell lymphoma, not otherwise specified (HGBL-NOS)	DLBCL arising from follicular lymphoma (FL) or marginal zone lymphoma (MZL)
HGBL with MYC and *BCL6* rearrangements (ICC)	Primary DLBCL of the central nervous system
Follicular lymphoma grade 3B (FL3B)/FLBCL	Richter transformation (DLBCL arising from chronic lymphocytic leukemia)

2 Testing for DLBCL » General health tests

General health tests

Some general health tests are described next. Tests to plan treatment can be found in **Guide 2.**

Medical history

A medical history is a record of all health issues and treatments you have had in your life. Be prepared to list any illness or injury and when it happened. Bring a list of old and new medicines and any over-the-counter (OTC) medicines, herbals, or supplements you take. Some supplements interact with and affect

Guide 2
Tests to plan treatment

Biopsy and pathology review

Biomarker testing with immunophenotyping and genetic mutation testing

Physical exam with special attention to lymph node-bearing areas (including Waldeyer's ring) and to size of liver and spleen

Performance status (PS)

B symptoms (fever, drenching night sweats, and loss of more than 10 percent of body weight over 6 months)

Complete blood count (CBC) with differential, lactate dehydrogenase (LDH), comprehensive metabolic panel (CMP), uric acid, and hepatitis B testing

PET/CT scan (preferred) or CT with contrast of chest, abdomen, and pelvis (C/A/P)

Heart tests

Calculation of International Prognostic Index (IPI), which predicts overall and progression-free survival in DLBCL based on risk factors

Pregnancy test for those of childbearing age if chemotherapy or radiation therapy will be used

Possible:
- Head or neck CT or MRI with contrast
- HIV testing
- Hepatitis C testing
- Beta-2-microglobulin
- Lumbar puncture for those at risk for central nervous system (CNS) involvement
- Bone marrow biopsy with or without aspirate
- Discussion of fertility preservation

medicines that your care team may prescribe. Tell your care team about any symptoms you have. A medical history, sometimes called a health history, will help determine which treatment is best for you.

Family history

Your care team will ask about the health history of family members who are blood relatives. This information is called a family history. Ask family members on both sides of your family about their health issues like heart disease, cancer, and diabetes, and at what age they were diagnosed. It's important to know the specific type of cancer or where the cancer started, if it is in multiple locations, and if they had genetic testing.

Physical exam

During a physical exam, a health care provider may:

- Check your temperature, blood pressure, pulse, and breathing rate
- Check your height and weight
- Listen to the lungs and heart
- Look in the eyes, ears, nose, and throat
- Feel and apply pressure to parts of your body to see if organs are of normal size, are soft or hard, or cause pain when touched.
- Feel for enlarged lymph nodes in the neck, underarm, and groin.

Fertility (all genders)

Treatment with targeted therapy and other forms of systemic (drug) therapy can affect your fertility, or the ability to have children. If you think you want children in the future, ask your care team how cancer and cancer treatment might affect your fertility.

Fertility preservation is all about keeping your options open, whether you know you want to have children later in life or aren't sure at the moment. Fertility and reproductive specialists can help you sort through what may be best for your situation.

More information on fertility preservation can be found in the *NCCN Guidelines for Patients: Adolescent and Young Adult Cancer* at NCCN.org/patientguidelines and on the NCCN Patient Guides for Cancer app.

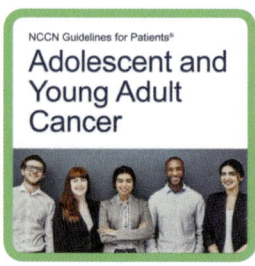

Changes in fertility

Treatment might cause your fertility to be temporarily or permanently impaired or interrupted. This loss of fertility is related to your age at time of diagnosis, treatment type(s), treatment dose, and treatment length. Talk to your care team about your concerns and if you are planning a pregnancy.

Preventing pregnancy during treatment

Cancer and cancer treatment can affect the ovaries and damage sperm. If you become pregnant during chemotherapy, radiation therapy, or other types of systemic therapy, serious birth defects can occur. Speak with your care team about preventing pregnancy while being treated for cancer. Hormonal birth control may or may not be recommended, so ask your doctor about options such as intrauterine devices (IUDs) and barrier methods. Types of barrier methods include condoms, diaphragms, cervical caps, and the contraceptive sponge.

Performance status

Performance status (PS) is a person's general level of fitness and ability to perform daily tasks. Your state of general health will be rated using a PS scale called the Eastern Cooperative Oncology Group (ECOG) score or the Karnofsky Performance Status (KPS). PS is one factor taken into consideration when choosing a treatment plan to ensure that the treatments your doctor recommends are safe for you. Your preferences about treatment are always important.

Blood tests

Blood tests check for signs of disease and how well organs are working. They require a sample of blood, which is removed through a needle placed into a vein in your arm. Be prepared to have many blood tests during DLBCL treatment and recovery to check treatment results, blood counts, and the health of organs like your liver and kidneys.

> **Information on possible tests and procedures can be found in this chapter. You do not need to know what all of these tests mean. It is okay to skip over information that doesn't interest you.**

Some possible blood tests are described next. They are listed alphabetically and not in order of importance.

Complete blood count and differential

A complete blood count (CBC) measures the levels of red blood cells (RBCs), white blood cells (WBCs), and platelets (PLTs) in your blood. A CBC is a key test that gives a picture of your overall health. A differential counts the number of each type of WBC (neutrophils, lymphocytes, monocytes, eosinophils, and basophils). It also checks if the counts are in balance with each other. Your doctor will likely pay most attention to the total white blood cell count, neutrophil count, hemoglobin, and platelets.

Comprehensive metabolic panel

A comprehensive metabolic panel (CMP) measures substances in your blood. It provides important information about how well your kidneys and liver are working, among other things.

2 Testing for DLBCL » Blood tests

Creatinine

Creatinine is a waste produced in the muscles. Every person generates a fixed amount of creatinine every day based on how much muscle they have. It is filtered out of the blood by the kidneys. The level of creatinine in the blood tells how well the kidneys are working. Higher levels of creatinine mean the kidneys aren't working as well as they were when someone had lower levels of creatinine.

Electrolytes

Electrolytes help move nutrients into cells and help move waste out of cells. Electrolytes are ions or particles with electrical charges that help the nerves, muscles, heart, and brain work as they should. Your body needs electrolytes to function properly.

Hepatitis B and hepatitis C

Hepatitis B (HBV) and hepatitis C (HCV) are types of virus infections that affect the liver. A hepatitis blood test will show if you had hepatitis in the past or if you have it today. Some cancer treatments can wake up (or reactivate) the virus. If this happens, it can cause harm to the liver.

HIV

Human immunodeficiency virus (HIV) weakens the immune system, increasing the risk of many cancers, and may cause acquired immunodeficiency syndrome (AIDS). An HIV antibody test checks for HIV antibodies in a sample of blood. It's important to let your doctor know if you have ever been infected with HIV. HIV screening is recommended for those with a new lymphoma diagnosis.

> **Testing takes time. It might take days or weeks for all test results to come in.**

HLA typing

Human leukocyte antigen (HLA) is a protein found on the surface of most cells. It plays an important role in your body's immune response. HLAs are unique to each person. They mark your body's cells. Your body detects these markers to tell which cells are yours. In other words, all your cells have the same set of HLAs called the HLA type or tissue type.

HLA typing is a blood test that detects a person's HLA type. This test is only done before a donor (allogeneic) hematopoietic cell transplant (HCT). An HCT is not common in DLBCL. To find a donor match, your proteins will be compared to the donor's proteins to see how many proteins are the same. Blood or tissue samples from you and your blood relatives will be tested first.

Lactate dehydrogenase

Lactate dehydrogenase (LDH) or lactic acid dehydrogenase is an enzyme found in most cells. Dying cells release LDH into blood. Fast-growing cells, such as tumor cells, also release LDH. Fast-growing cells also release LDH and cause levels of this protein to be elevated in the blood.

Pregnancy test

If planned treatment might affect pregnancy, then those who can become pregnant will be given a pregnancy test before treatment begins.

SPEP

Serum protein electrophoresis (SPEP) examines specific proteins in the blood called globulins, which may be increased in certain conditions.

Uric acid

Uric acid is released by cells when DNA breaks down. It is a normal waste product that dissolves in your blood and is filtered by the kidneys where it leaves the body as urine. Too much uric acid in the body is called hyperuricemia. With DLBCL, it can be caused by a fast turnover of lymphoma cells. High uric acid might be a side effect of chemotherapy or radiation therapy. Very high levels of uric acid in the blood can damage the kidneys.

Biopsy

A biopsy is the removal of tissue or fluid for testing. It is an important part of an accurate diagnosis of lymphoma. Your sample should be reviewed by a pathologist who is an expert in the diagnosis of lymphoma. The pathologist will note the overall appearance and the size, shape, and type of your cells. This review is often referred to as histology, histopathology, or hematopathology review. Tests will be done on the biopsied cells. Ask questions about your biopsy results and what they mean for your treatment.

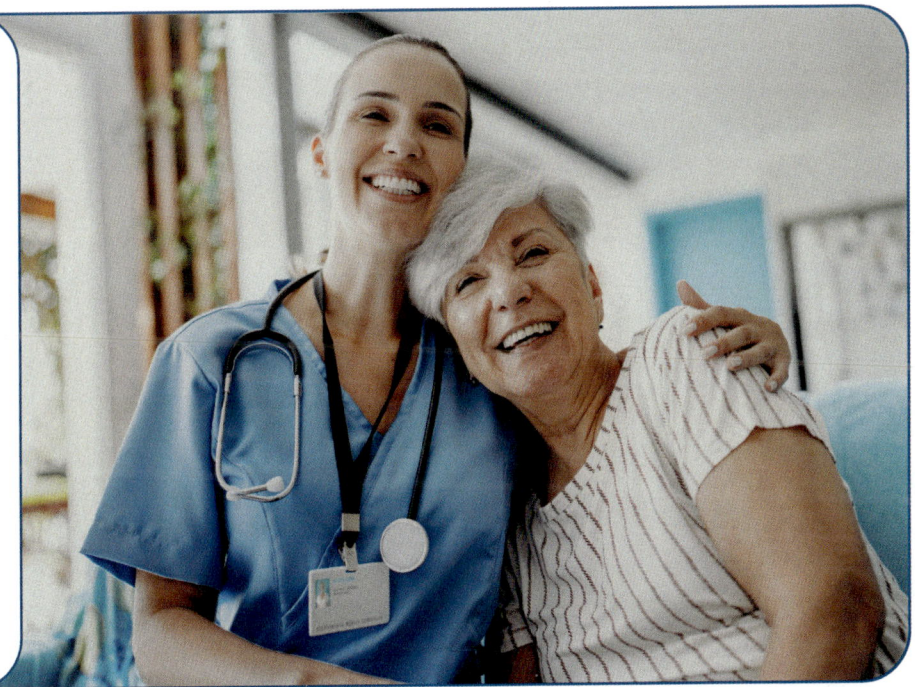

"I was so fortunate to find an expert oncologist and health care team that I could openly and honestly talk to during and after my treatment. This resulted in shared decision-making over my care. I credit this to my being here 35 years later."

2 Testing for DLBCL » Immunophenotyping

Types of possible biopsies include the following:

> **Fine-needle aspiration (FNA) and core biopsy (CB)** use needles of different sizes to remove a sample of tissue or fluid.

> **Incisional biopsy** removes a small amount of tissue through a cut in the skin or body.

> **Excisional biopsy** removes the entire tumor through a cut in the skin or body.

> **Lymph node biopsy** removes tissue from a lymph node.

A biopsy is usually done with other lab methods to accurately diagnose the type of DLBCL. When possible, larger tissue samples obtained through excisional, incisional, or lymph node biopsies are often preferred for diagnosing DLBCL.

Lymph node biopsy

A lymph node biopsy may be needed to diagnose DLBCL. Lymph nodes are usually too small to be seen or felt. Sometimes, lymph nodes can feel swollen, enlarged, hard to the touch, or don't move when pushed (fixed or immobile). A lymph node biopsy can be done using a needle biopsy procedure or as a small surgery to remove (excise) a lymph node.

Bone marrow tests

Bone marrow tests might be done in certain cases. There are 2 types of bone marrow tests that are often done at the same time:

> Bone marrow aspirate

> Bone marrow biopsy

Bone marrow aspirate and biopsy are bedside procedures. It is not surgery and does not require an operating room. Your care team will try to make you as comfortable as possible during the procedure. The samples are usually taken from the back of the hip bone (pelvis). You will likely lie on your belly or side. For an aspirate, a hollow needle will be pushed through your skin and into the bone. Liquid bone marrow will then be drawn into a syringe. For the biopsy, a wider needle will be used to remove a small piece of bone. You may feel bone pain at your hip for a few days. Your skin may bruise.

Immunophenotyping

Immunophenotyping is a process that uses antibodies to detect the presence or absence of certain antigens. Antigens are proteins or markers that can be found on the surface of or inside all cells, including white blood cells. Specific groupings of antigens are normal. However, some specific patterns of antigens called the immunophenotype are found on abnormal cells including non-Hodgkin lymphoma (NHL) and DLBCL.

Immunophenotyping can be done using specialized techniques called flow cytometry or immunohistochemistry. These techniques are used to distinguish DLBCL from other types of

2 Testing for DLBCL » Immunophenotyping

lymphoma. Immunophenotype can change as cancer progresses.

Immunophenotyping is used to help support a diagnosis. However, an accurate diagnosis requires a trained pathologist to review the tissue for abnormal cells seen under a microscope. More testing may be needed to establish a subtype.

DLBCL is divided into 2 broad categories:

- Germinal center B-cell (GCB)
- Non-GCB

Immunophenotyping is used to establish diagnosis and GCB versus non-GCB origin. **See Guide 3**.

Flow cytometry

Flow cytometry is a lab method used to detect, identify, and count specific cells. Flow cytometry involves adding a light-sensitive dye to cells. The dyed cells are passed through a beam of light in a machine. The machine measures the number of cells, things like the size and shape of the cells.

Flow cytometry may be used on cells from circulating (peripheral) blood or from a bone marrow aspirate. A blood test can count the number of white blood cells, but it cannot detect the subtle differences between different types of blood cancers. Flow cytometry can detect these subtle differences. The most common use of flow cytometry is in the identification of markers on cells, particularly in the immune system (called immunophenotyping).

Guide 3
Tests to diagnose DLBCL

Needed	• Biopsy and hematopathology review • Immunohistochemistry (IHC) panel: CD3, CD20, CD10, CD21, BCL2, BCL6, IRF4/MUM1, and MYC with or without cell surface marker analysis by flow cytometry: kappa/ lambda, CD3, CD5, CD19, CD10, CD20, and CD45 • Karyotype or fluorescence in situ hybridization (FISH) for *MYC* • FISH for *BCL2* and *BCL6* rearrangements if *MYC* positive
In some cases	• Additional IHC studies to determine LBCL subtype: cyclin D1, kappa/lambda, CD5, CD30, CD45, CD138, anaplastic lymphoma kinase (ALK), human herpesvirus-8 (HHV8), SOX11, and Ki-67 • Epstein-Barr encoding region in situ hybridization (EBER-ISH) • Karyotype or FISH for *IRF4/MUM1* rearrangements • Next-generation sequencing (NGS) lymphoma panel

Immunohistochemistry

Immunohistochemistry (IHC) is a special staining process that involves adding a chemical marker to cells. The cells are then studied using a microscope. IHC looks for the immunophenotype of cells from a biopsy or tissue sample.

Testing for DLBCL biomarker and genetic changes

Biomarker and genetic tests are used to learn more about your type of DLBCL, to guide treatment, and to determine the likely path your cancer will take (prognosis). This genetic testing is different from family history genetic testing or genetic cancer risk testing. This testing looks for changes only in the DLBCL cells that have developed over time, and not changes in the rest of the body's cells. It is sometimes called molecular testing, tumor profiling, gene expression profiling, or genomic testing.

Inside our cells are DNA (deoxyribonucleic acid) molecules. These molecules are tightly packaged into what is called a chromosome. Chromosomes contain most of the genetic information in a cell. Normal human cells contain 23 pairs of chromosomes for a total of 46 chromosomes. Each chromosome contains thousands of genes. Genes are coded instructions for the proteins your cells make. A mutation is when something goes wrong in the genetic code. Proteins are written like this: BCL6. Genes are written with italics like this: *BCL6*. When a gene or protein is found (expressed), it is shown with a plus sign (+)

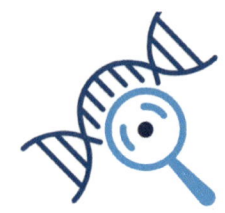

DLBCL genetic changes

DLBCL cells can have changes in genes and chromosomes. Mutation testing looks for these changes or abnormalities that are unique to DLBCL cells. Examples of such changes are called deletion, inversion, insertion, amplification, translocation (rearrangement), and point mutation.

- **Amplification** – When part of or a whole chromosome or gene is increased (for example, duplicated)
- **Deletion** – When part of a chromosome or gene is missing
- **Insertion** – When a new part of a chromosome or gene is included
- **Inversion** – Switching of parts within 1 chromosome
- **Point mutation** – When part of a gene is changed
- **Chromosome translocation and gene rearrangement** – Switching of parts between 2 chromosomes. When described at the chromosome level, it is called a translocation. When described at the gene level, it is called rearrangement.

2 Testing for DLBCL » Testing for DLBCL biomarker and genetic changes

like this: CD10+. When a gene or protein has not been found, it is written with a negative sign (-) like this CD10-.

DLBCL cells sometimes have changes in genes and chromosomes that can be seen under a microscope or found with other tests.

> Testing of your lymphoma cells can gather specific information about your lymphoma to help guide treatment.

Beta-2-microglobulin tumor marker test

Beta-2-microglobulin (B2M) is a protein that can be found in the blood, urine, or cerebrospinal fluid (CSF). B2M is a type of tumor marker. Tumor markers are substances made by cancer cells or by normal cells in response to cancer in the body.

Epstein-Barr virus in situ hybridization

Epstein-Barr encoding region (EBER) in situ hybridization (EBER-ISH) is used to detect the Epstein-Barr virus (EBV) in tissue samples. EBV sometimes can be found in those with DLBCL. This test can help determine the subtype of DLBCL.

DLBCL mutation testing

A sample of your blood or bone marrow may be used to see if the DLBCL cancer cells have any specific mutations. Lymph nodes and other tissues can also analyzed for mutations. Some mutations can be targeted with specific therapies. This is separate from the genetic testing for mutations that you may have inherited from your biological parents.

Mutation testing includes tests of genes or their products (proteins). Subtle new drug-resistant mutations may occur over time. Mutations can also happen during treatment. Mutation testing is used to look for these new mutations. Some mutations lead to resistance to certain targeted therapies. There are many possible mutations.

Gene rearrangements

In gene rearrangements, part of a gene has broken off and attached to another gene, creating a new gene. When one cell divides many times, the entire group of cells is called clonal or clonality. In clonal rearrangements, the same gene rearrangements are found in a group of cancer cells.

> *MYC*, *BCL2*, and *BCL6* gene rearrangements are commonly found in DLBCL.

MYC

The gene for *MYC* (proto-oncogene) is found on chromosome 8. An *MYC* gene rearrangement (*MYC*-R) is often found with a *BCL2* or *BCL6* gene rearrangement.

BCL2

The gene for *BCL2* (B-cell lymphoma 2) is found on chromosome 18. The transfer of the *BCL2* gene to a different chromosome causes the BCL2 protein to be made in larger amounts, which may keep cancer cells from dying.

BCL6

The gene for *BCL6* (B-cell lymphoma 6) is found on chromosome 3. *BCL6* rearrangement is the most frequent chromosomal abnormality found in DLBCL.

Deletions

When part of a chromosome is missing, it is called a deletion. For example, in del(7q) the q part of chromosome 7 is missing (deleted). Specific chromosomal deletions can be found in some types of diffuse B-cell lymphomas but can also be found in other types of blood cancers and disorders.

FISH

Fluorescence in situ hybridization (FISH) is a method that involves special dyes called probes that attach to pieces of DNA. Since this test doesn't need growing cells, it can be performed on bone marrow or a blood sample.

FISH can find translocations that are too small to be seen with other methods. A translocation occurs when parts of two chromosomes switch with one another. However, FISH can only be used for known changes. It cannot detect all the possible changes found within the chromosomes and genes. For example, FISH is used to detect *MYC*, *BCL2*, and *BCL6* gene rearrangements.

Karyotype

A karyotype is a picture of chromosomes. Normal human cells contain 23 pairs of chromosomes for a total of 46 chromosomes. A karyotype will show extra, missing, rearranged, or abnormal pieces of chromosomes. Since a karyotype requires growing cells, a sample of bone marrow or blood must be used.

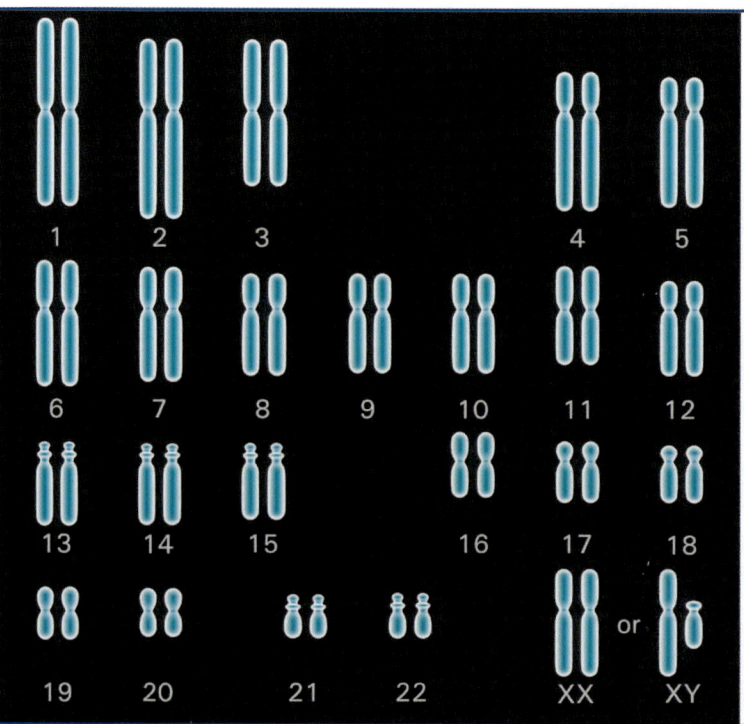

Karyotype

A karyotype is a picture of your chromosomes. The study of chromosomes is called cytogenetics.

Translocations

Translocation is a switching of parts between two chromosomes. A translocation between chromosomes 11 and 18 is written as t(11;18). Specific translocations can help distinguish between types of blood cancers and disorders.

PCR

A polymerase chain reaction (PCR) is a technique that can make millions or billions of copies of your DNA or RNA (genetic information). PCR is very sensitive. It can find 1 abnormal cell among more than 100,000 normal cells. These copies, called PCR products, might be used for NGS. This is important when testing for treatment response or remission.

Comparative genomic hybridization

Comparative genomic hybridization (CGH) is a technique that compares DNA samples from normal tissue and tumor tissue. It is used to detect abnormal chromosomes.

High-throughput sequencing

High-throughput sequencing (HTS) is capable of sequencing hundreds of millions of DNA molecules at a time.

Next-generation sequencing

Next-generation sequencing (NGS) is a method used to determine a portion of a person's DNA sequence. It shows if a gene has any mutations that might affect how the gene works. NGS looks at the gene in a more detailed way than other methods and can find mutations that other methods might miss.

Genetic cancer risk testing

Genetic cancer risk testing is done using blood or saliva (spitting into a cup or cheek swab). The goal is to look for gene mutations inherited from your biological parents called germline mutations. Some mutations can put you at risk for more than one type of cancer. You can pass these genes on to your children. Also, family members might carry these mutations. Tell your care team if there is a family history of cancer.

Imaging tests

Imaging tests take pictures of the inside of your body to look for cancer deposits. A radiologist, an expert in interpreting imaging tests, will write a report and send this report to your doctor. While these reports might be available to you through your patient portal or patient access system, please wait to discuss these results with your care team.

Contrast material

Contrast materials are substances that help enhance and improve the images of several organs and structures in the body. It is used to make the pictures clearer. The types of contrast vary and are different for CT and MRI. Not all imaging tests require contrast, but many do.

Tell the care team if you have had allergic reactions to contrast in the past. This is important. You might be given medicines to avoid the effects of those allergies. Contrast might not be used if you have a serious allergy or if your kidneys aren't working well.

CT scan

A computed tomography (CT or CAT) scan uses x-rays and computer technology to take pictures of the inside of the body. It takes many x-rays of the same body part from different angles. All the images are combined to make one detailed picture. A CT scan of your head, neck, chest abdomen, and pelvis may be one of the tests to look for cancer. In most cases, contrast will be used.

MRI scan

A magnetic resonance imaging (MRI) scan uses radio waves and powerful magnets to take pictures of the inside of the body. It does not use x-rays. Because of the very strong magnets used in the MRI machine, tell the technologist if you have any metal in your body. During the test, you will likely be asked to hold your breath for 10 to 20 seconds as the technician collects the images. Contrast is often used.

A closed MRI has a capsule-like design where the magnet surrounds you. The space is small and enclosed. An open MRI has a magnetic top and bottom, which allows for an opening on each end. Closed MRIs are more common than open MRIs, so if you have claustrophobia (a dread or fear of enclosed spaces), be sure to talk to your care team about it.

PET scan

A PET (positron emission tomography) scan uses a radioactive drug called a tracer. A tracer is a substance injected into a vein to see where cancer cells are in the body and how much sugar is being taken up by the cancer cells. This gives an idea about how fast the

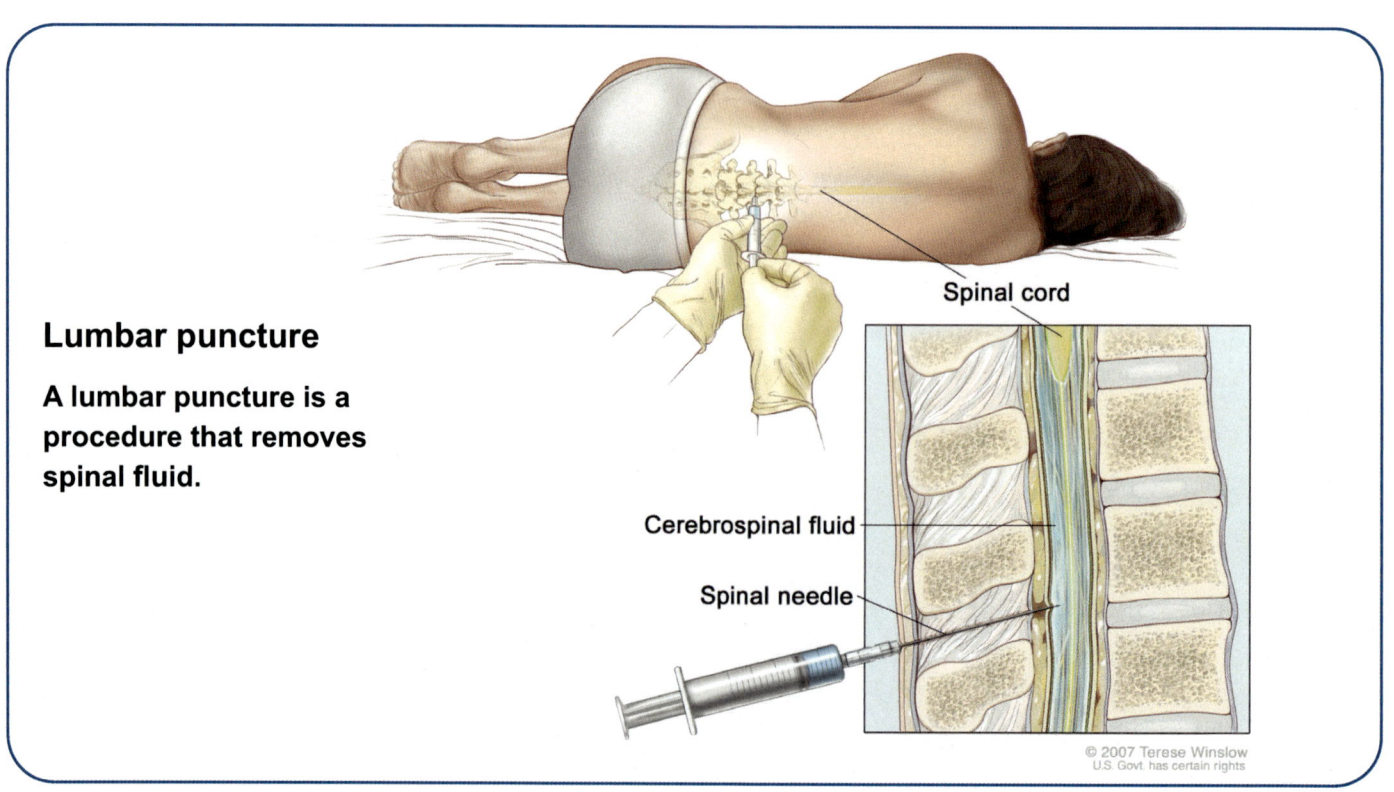

Lumbar puncture

A lumbar puncture is a procedure that removes spinal fluid.

cancer cells are growing. Cancer cells show up as bright spots on PET scans. However, not all tumors will appear on a PET scan. Also, not all bright spots found on the PET scan are cancer. It is normal for the brain, heart, kidneys, and bladder to be bright on PET. Inflammation or infection can also show up as a bright spot. When a PET scan is combined with CT, it is called a PET/CT scan. An FDG-PET/CT uses a radiotracer called fluorodeoxyglucose (FDG). You will be asked to not eat (fast) for a number of hours before the scan. You can eat and drink normally after the test is completed.

Scrotal ultrasound

DLBCL can occasionally be found in the testicles. A scrotal ultrasound uses sound waves to make images of the scrotum. The scrotum is the pouch of skin at the base of the penis that contains the testicles.

Lumbar puncture

Lymphoma can travel to the fluid that surrounds the spine or brain. This may cause symptoms such as headaches, neck pain, and sensitivity to light. To know if lymphoma cells are in your central nervous system (CNS), a sample of spinal fluid must be taken and tested. A lumbar puncture (LP) is a procedure that removes spinal fluid. It is also called a spinal tap. A lumbar puncture may also be used to inject cancer drugs into spinal fluid. This is called intrathecal (IT) chemotherapy. When systemic therapy and IT therapy are given together to prevent CNS disease, it is called CNS prophylaxis.

Heart tests

Heart or cardiac tests are used to see how well the heart works. These tests are performed prior to the start of treatment and might be used to monitor treatment side effects. You might be referred to a heart specialist called a cardiologist.

Electrocardiogram

An electrocardiogram (ECG or EKG) shows electrical changes in your heart. It reveals information about your heart rate and rhythm. A prolonged corrected QT interval (or QTc) occurs when your heart muscle takes longer than normal to recharge between beats. Certain treatments can cause a prolonged QTc. If the QTc becomes too prolonged, it can cause dangerous heart rhythms.

Echocardiogram

An echocardiogram (or echo) uses sound waves to make pictures. It is a type of ultrasound. For this test, small patches will be placed on your chest to track your heartbeat. Next, a wand with gel on its tip will be slid across part of your bare chest. A picture of your beating heart will be seen on a screen. The pictures will be recorded for future viewing.

An echocardiogram shows the structure (valves and muscle thickness) and function of your heart (or ejection fraction). Ejection fraction is the amount of blood pumped out of the left side of your heart every time it beats. If the amount of blood pumping from the left side of the heart is lower than normal, this indicates decreased heart function.

2 Testing for DLBCL » Key points » Questions to ask

Key points

- In diffuse large B-cell lymphoma (DLBCL), tumors of fast-growing, large B-cell lymphocytes, a type of white blood cell, are commonly found in lymph nodes, spleen, liver, bone marrow, or other tissues and organs.

- A biopsy is the removal of tissue or fluid for testing. It is an important part of an accurate DLBCL diagnosis.

- Genetic and biomarker tests are used to learn more about your subtype of DLBCL, to target treatment, and to determine the likely course the cancer will take called a prognosis.

- Immunophenotyping is used to diagnose and pinpoint the specific subtype of DLBCL.

- *MYC*, *BCL2*, and *BCL6* are gene rearrangements that might be found in DLBCL.

- Imaging tests are used to look for areas of lymphoma involvement and are part of your staging workup.

- A lumbar puncture (LP) may be done to look for DLBCL in spinal and brain fluid.

Questions to ask

- What subtype of DLBCL do I have? What does this mean in terms of prognosis and treatment options?

- Is there a cancer center or hospital nearby that specializes in my subtype of lymphoma?

- What tests will I have? How often will they be repeated?

- Will my insurance pay for these tests?

- Who will talk with me about the next steps? When?

3
Types of treatment

26 Care team

26 Treatment phases

28 Systemic therapy

28 Chemotherapy

29 Chemoimmunotherapy

29 Immunotherapy

31 Other systemic therapies

31 Targeted therapy

31 Radiation therapy

32 Hematopoietic cell transplant

33 Surgery

34 Clinical trials

35 Key points

35 Questions to ask

3 Types of treatment » Care team » Treatment phases

There is more than one treatment for diffuse large B-cell lymphomas. This chapter presents an overview of the possible types of treatment and what to expect. Not everyone will receive the same treatment. Treatment options are based on many factors. Together, you and your care team will choose a treatment plan that is best for you.

Diffuse large B-cell lymphoma (DLBCL) is highly treatable. The goal of treatment is to cure the disease. For many people with DLBCL, treatment is usually a combination of chemotherapy and immunotherapy called chemoimmunotherapy. Radiation therapy might be added. Surgery is not a routine part of treatment for DLBCL.

It is important to have regular talks with your care team about your goals for treatment and your treatment plan.

Care team

Treating DLBCL takes a team approach. Treatment decisions should involve a multidisciplinary team (MDT). An MDT is a team of health care and psychosocial care professionals from different professional backgrounds who have knowledge (expertise) and experience in your type of cancer.

This team is united in the planning and implementing of your treatment. Ask who will coordinate your care.

Some members of your care team will be with you throughout cancer treatment, while others will only be there for parts of it. Get to know your care team and help them get to know you.

Your team might include the following specialists:

> - **A hematologist or hematologic oncologist** is a medical expert in blood diseases and blood cancers and uses systemic (drug) therapy to treat these conditions.
> - **A radiation oncologist** prescribes and plans radiation therapy to treat cancer.
> - **A pathologist or hematopathologist** analyzes the cells and tissues removed during a biopsy and provides cancer diagnosis and information about biomarker testing.

Treatment phases

The goal of treatment is remission. Here are some terms you might hear used by your care team.

Induction

Induction or first-line therapy is the first phase of treatment. The goal of induction is complete response (CR) or complete remission. After induction, you will have tests to look for a response (remission).

Remission

There are different types of treatment response. When there are no signs of cancer, it is called a complete response (CR) or complete remission. Remission can be short-term (temporary) or long-lasting (permanent). In partial response (PR), cancer is still present, but it has reduced in size or amount.

Relapse

When DLBCL returns after a period of remission, it is called a relapse. The goal of treatment is to achieve remission again. A relapse is very serious. It is important to ask about your prognosis.

Refractory

When DLBCL remains and does not respond to treatment, it is called refractory or resistant cancer. This cancer may be resistant at the start of treatment or it may become resistant during treatment. Refractory disease is very serious. It is important to ask about your prognosis.

Surveillance and monitoring

You will be monitored throughout treatment. Surveillance watches for any changes in your condition after completing treatment. You will have tests during surveillance to check for relapse.

Standard of care is the best-known way to treat a particular disease based on past clinical trials. There may be more than one treatment regimen that is considered standard of care. Ask your care team what treatment options are available and if a clinical trial might be right for you.

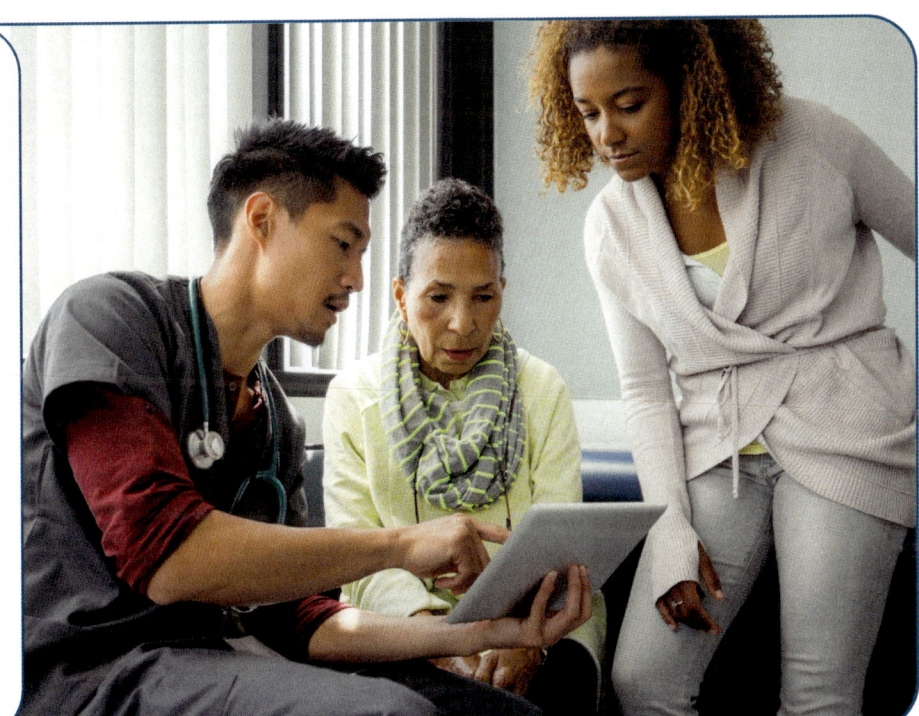

Systemic therapy

Systemic therapy works throughout the body. Types include chemotherapy, chemoimmunotherapy, immunotherapy, and targeted therapy. Systemic therapy might be used alone or with other therapies. Goals of systemic therapy may be curative or palliative and should be discussed before starting treatment.

The choice of therapy takes into consideration many factors, including age, other serious health issues, and future treatment possibilities like a hematopoietic cell transplant (HCT). Your preferences about treatment are important. If you have any religious or personal beliefs about certain kinds of treatment, now would be the time to share them with your care team.

Treatment options

Treatment options are often described in the following ways:

- **Preferred therapies** have the most evidence they work better and may be safer than other therapies.

- **Other recommended therapies** may not work quite as well as preferred therapies, but they can still help treat cancer.

- **Therapies used in certain cases** work best for people with specific cancer features or health circumstances.

Chemotherapy

Chemotherapy kills fast-dividing cells throughout the body, including cancer cells and some normal cells. More than one chemotherapy may be used to treat DLBCL. When only one drug is used, it's called a single agent. A combination or multi-agent regimen is the use of two or more cancer-fighting drugs.

Some chemotherapy drugs are liquids that are infused into a vein or injected under the skin with a needle. Other chemotherapy drugs may be given as a pill that is swallowed. The final dose often differs between people because doses may be based on body weight and height. Intrathecal (IT) chemotherapy is injected into the fluid surrounding the brain and spinal cord.

In most cases, chemotherapy is given in cycles of treatment days followed by days of rest. This allows the body to recover before the next cycle. Cycles vary in length depending on which chemotherapy is used. You will have tests to see how the cancer is responding to treatment. You might spend time in the hospital during treatment.

Here are 2 examples of a chemotherapy drug combination (regimen):

- **CHOP** – Cyclophosphamide, doxorubicin, vincristine, and prednisone

- **EPOCH** – Etoposide (Etopophos), prednisone, vincristine, cyclophosphamide, and doxorubicin

Chemoimmunotherapy

Chemoimmunotherapy, also called immunochemotherapy, includes chemotherapy and immunotherapy drugs (agents) to treat cancer. There are several chemoimmunotherapy regimens used to treat DLBCL.

Two examples include:

> **RCHOP** – Rituximab, cyclophosphamide (Cytoxan), doxorubicin, vincristine (Oncovin), and prednisone

> **Pola-R-CHP** – Polatuzumab vedotin-piiq (Polivy), rituximab, cyclophosphamide, doxorubicin, and prednisone

CD19-targeting CAR T-cell therapy

CAR T-cell therapy is made by removing T cells from your body and then engineering your own immune cells to fight the lymphoma for you by adding a CAR (chimeric antigen receptor) to the T cells. This programs the T cells to find cancer cells. The programmed T cells will be infused back into your body to find and kill cancer cells. This treatment is not for everyone.

CAR T-cell therapy is one way to target the CD19 protein found on almost at B-cell lymphomas, including DLBCL. CAR T-cell therapy is only used in recurrent lymphoma outside of clinical trials.

CD19-directed CAR T-cell therapy options for DLBCL include axicabtagene ciloleucel (Yescarta), lisocabtagene maraleucel (Breyanzi), and tisagenlecleucel (Kymriah).

For more information on CAR T-cell therapy, see *NCCN Guidelines for Patients:*

Immunotherapy Side Effects at NCCN.org/patientguidelines and on the NCCN Patient Guides for Cancer app.

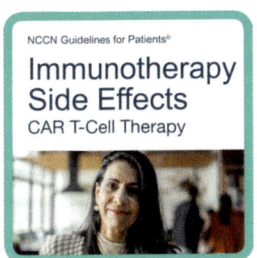

Immunotherapy

Immunotherapy is drug therapy that helps your immune system better identify and destroy cancer cells. By doing so, it improves your body's ability to find and destroy cancer cells. Immunotherapy can be given alone or with other types of treatment.

Antibody therapy

Antibody therapy uses antibodies to help the body fight cancer, infection, or other diseases. Antibodies are proteins made by the immune system that bind to specific markers on cells or tissues. A monoclonal antibody is made from a unique white blood cell, such as B or plasma cell. Monoclonal antibodies (mAbs) used in cancer treatment may kill cancer cells directly, block development of tumor blood vessels, or help the immune system kill cancer cells. As with other treatments, there is the potential for complications.

CD19-targeting monoclonal antibody therapy

Tafasitamab-cxix (Monjuvi) is used to treat DLBCL by targeting the CD19 protein.

3 Types of treatment » Immunotherapy

CD20-targeting monoclonal antibody therapy

CD20-targeting mAbs (also called anti-CD20 mAbs) such as rituximab (Rituxan) and obinutuzumab (Gazyva) target the CD20 protein found on the surface of B cells and DLBCL. The drug attaches to the CD20 protein alerting the immune system to the cancer. This triggers normal immune cells to kill the cancer cells.

Bispecific antibody therapy

Bispecific antibodies (BsAbs) bind to 2 different proteins (CD20 and CD3 antigen) at the same time. It treats cancer by engaging and activating T cells and redirecting them to the site of the lymphoma. Bispecific examples include epcoritamab-bysp (Epkinly), mosunetuzumab-axgb (Lunsumio), and glofitamab-gxbm (Columvi). Bispecifics can cause a side effect called cytokine release syndrome (CRS).

PD-1-targeting monoclonal antibody therapy

Pembrolizumab (Keytruda) and nivolumab (Opdivo) with or without brentuximab vedotin (an antibody drug conjugate) might be used to treat relapsed or refractory primary mediastinal large B-cell lymphoma. These drugs block the ability of cancer cells to hide from your body's immune system.

Warnings about supplements and drug interactions

You might be asked to stop taking or avoid certain herbal supplements when on a systemic therapy. Some supplements can affect the ability of a drug to do its job. This is called a drug interaction.

It is critical to speak with your care team about any supplements you may be taking. Some examples include:

- Turmeric
- Ginkgo biloba
- Green tea extract
- St. John's Wort
- Antioxidants

Certain medicines can also affect the ability of a drug to do its job. Antacids, heart or blood pressure medicine, and antidepressants are just some of the medicines that might interact with a systemic therapy or supportive care medicines given during systemic therapy. Therefore, it is very important to tell your care team about any medicines, vitamins, over-the-counter (OTC) drugs, herbals, or supplements you are taking.

Bring a list with you to every visit. Tell your care team about any changes in your medicines.

Other systemic therapies

Antibody drug conjugate

An antibody drug conjugate (ADC) delivers cell-specific chemotherapy. It attaches to a protein found on the outside of the cancer cell and then enters the cell. Once inside the cell, chemotherapy is released. Loncastuximab tesirine-lpyl (Zynlonta) is an ADC that targets the CD19 protein. Polatuzumab vedotin-piiq targets the CD79b protein and brentuximab vedotin targets the CD30 protein.

Enzyme inhibitor

A topoisomerase inhibitor blocks enzymes involved in cell division. Etoposide (Etopophos) is one example. A topoisomerase enzyme inhibitor may be used with other types of chemotherapy.

Immune modulator

An immune modulator changes your immune system so it can target cancer cells more effectively. Lenalidomide (Revlimid) is an example of an immune modulator.

Targeted therapy

Targeted therapy is drug therapy that focuses on specific or unique features of cancer cells. Targeted therapies seek out how cancer cells grow, divide, and move in the body. These drugs stop or inhibit the action of molecules that help cancer cells grow and/or survive.

> **A biosimilar or substitute might be used in place of rituximab.**
>
> A biosimilar is an almost identical version of a drug made by another company. It is used in the exact same way and at the same dose as rituximab. Biosimilars for rituximab include: Riabni, Hycela, Ruxience, and Truxima.

Some targeted therapy examples include:

- Alectinib (Alecensa) and lorlatinib (Lorbrena) target the activity of the ALK protein found in those with an *ALK* gene mutation.
- Ibrutinib (Imbruvica) is a Bruton tyrosine kinase inhibitor (BTKi). It blocks the BTK protein, which the cancer relies on for survival. Since a major signal for B cell growth is blocked, this can cause the lymphoma cells to eventually die off.

Radiation therapy

Radiation therapy (RT) uses high-energy radiation from photons, electrons, or protons, and other sources to kill cancer cells and shrink tumors. RT may be used as the main treatment to cure cancer (curative treatment), or as supportive care or palliative care to help ease pain or discomfort caused by cancer.

Radiation is typically delivered from outside the body by a computerized device, which can shape the treatment to closely fit the location and size of the tumor. Treatment is given in small daily doses on weekdays, with weekends off.

You will see your radiation oncologist at least weekly to review treatment results and to help with side effects, such as sunburn-like rash. Ask your care team which radiation option(s) are best for your situation, if RT will be combined with chemotherapy, and what side effects to expect. RT puts you at a small risk of developing other cancers in the future.

A four-dimensional (4D) CT scan might be used to plan RT. A 4D-CT records multiple images over time. It allows playback of the scan as a video, so that internal movement can be tracked and observed.

External beam radiation

External beam radiation therapy (EBRT) uses a machine outside of the body to aim radiation at the tumor(s) or areas of the body.

Common types of EBRT that may be used to treat your cancer include the following:

- **Three-dimensional conformal radiation therapy (3D-CRT)** uses computer software and CT images to aim beams that match the shape of the tumor.

- **Intensity-modulated radiation therapy (IMRT)** uses small beams of different strengths to match the shape of the tumor.

- **Involved-site radiation therapy (ISRT)** treats cancer found in a small region or one area of your body or cancer found in or near lymph nodes (nodal disease).

Hematopoietic cell transplant

A hematopoietic cell transplant (HCT) is a cancer treatment that replaces a person's bone marrow and immune system with donor cells to fight the lymphoma. An HCT replaces hematopoietic stem cells that have been destroyed by high doses of chemotherapy and/or radiation therapy as part of the transplant process. A hematopoietic stem cell is an immature cell that can develop into any type of blood cell. HCTs are performed in specialized centers.

There are 2 types of HCTs:

- **Autologous** – stem cells come from you. An autologous transplant is also called HDT/ASCR (high-dose therapy with autologous stem cell rescue) or an autologous HCT.

- **Allogeneic** – stem cells come from a donor who may or may not be related to you. Compared to an autologous HCT, an allogeneic HCT introduces new immune cells from the donor which may be able to detect and eliminate cancer cells better than your immune system was able to (known as graft-versus-lymphoma effect).

Conditioning

Before an HCT, treatment is needed to destroy bone marrow cells. This is called conditioning and it creates room for transplanted healthy stem cells. It also weakens the immune system so your body won't kill the transplanted cells. Chemotherapy is used for conditioning.

3 Types of treatment » Surgery

After conditioning, you will receive a transfusion of healthy stem cells. A transfusion is a slow injection of blood products into a vein. This can take several hours. The transplanted stem cells will travel to your bone marrow and grow. New, healthy blood cells will form. This is called engraftment. It usually takes about 2 to 4 weeks. Until then, you will have little or no immune defense. You may need to stay in a very clean room at the hospital or be given antibiotics to prevent or treat infection. Transfusions are also possible. A red blood cell transfusion is used to prevent bleeding and to treat anemia (below normal red blood cell count). A platelet transfusion is used to treat a low platelet count or bleeding. While waiting for the cells to engraft, you will likely feel tired and weak.

The goal of the transplant is for the new immune system to recognize the lymphoma as foreign and destroy it.

Possible side effects

Every treatment has side effects. You will be monitored for infections, disease relapse, and graft-versus-host disease (GVHD). In GVHD, the donor cells attack your normal, healthy tissue. There are treatments for GVHD. Ask the care team about the possible side effects or complications of HCT and how this might affect your quality of life.

More information on GVHD can be found in the *NCCN Guidelines for Patients: Graft-Versus-Host Disease* at NCCN.org/patientguidelines and on the NCCN Patient Guides for Cancer app.

Finding a clinical trial

In the United States

NCCN Cancer Centers
NCCN.org/cancercenters

The National Cancer Institute (NCI)
cancer.gov/about-cancer/treatment/clinical-trials/search

Worldwide

The U.S. National Library of Medicine (NLM)
clinicaltrials.gov/

Need help finding a clinical trial?

NCI's Cancer Information Service (CIS)
1.800.4.CANCER (1.800.422.6237)
cancer.gov/contact

Surgery

Surgery is an operation or procedure to remove cancer from the body. Surgery is not a routine part of treatment for DLBCL. If surgery is needed, seek the opinion of an experienced surgeon. Hospitals that perform many surgeries often have better results. You can ask for a referral to a hospital or cancer center that has experience in treating your type of cancer.

3 Types of treatment » Clinical trials

Clinical trials

A clinical trial is a type of medical research study. After being developed and tested in a lab, potential new ways of treating cancer need to be studied in people. If found to be safe and effective in a clinical trial, a drug, device, or treatment approach may be approved by the U.S. Food and Drug Administration (FDA).

Everyone with cancer should carefully consider all of the treatment options available for their cancer type, including standard treatments and clinical trials. Talk to your doctor about whether a clinical trial may make sense for you.

Phases

Most cancer clinical trials focus on treatment and are done in phases.

- **Phase 1** trials study the safety and side effects of an investigational drug or treatment approach.
- **Phase 2** trials study how well the drug or approach works against a specific type of cancer.
- **Phase 3** trials test the drug or approach against a standard treatment. If the results are good, it may be approved by the FDA.
- **Phase 4** trials study the safety and benefit of an FDA-approved treatment.

Who can enroll?

It depends on the clinical trial's rules, called eligibility criteria. The rules may be about age, cancer type and stage, treatment history, or general health. They ensure that participants are alike in specific ways and that the trial is as safe as possible for the participants.

Informed consent

Clinical trials are managed by a research team. This group of experts will review the study with you in detail, including its purpose and the risks and benefits of joining. All of this information is also provided in an informed consent form. Read the form carefully and ask questions before signing it. Take time to discuss the trial with people you trust. Keep in mind that you can leave and seek treatment outside of the clinical trial at any time.

Will I get a placebo?

Placebos (inactive versions of real medicines) are almost never used alone in cancer clinical trials. It is common to receive either a placebo with a standard treatment, or a new drug with a standard treatment. You will be informed, verbally and in writing, if a placebo is part of a clinical trial before you enroll.

Are clinical trials free?

There is no fee to enroll in a clinical trial. The study sponsor pays for research-related costs, including the study drug. But you may need to pay for other services, like transportation or childcare, due to extra appointments. During the trial, you will continue to receive standard cancer care. This care is often covered by insurance.

3 Types of treatment » Key points » Questions to ask

Key points

- Diffuse large B-cell lymphoma (DLBCL) is highly treatable. The goal of treatment is to cure the disease.

- Treatment can affect fertility in all sexes. Those who want to have children in the future should be referred to a fertility specialist before starting chemotherapy and/or radiation therapy to discuss the options.

- Systemic (drug) therapy works throughout the body. DLBCL is treated with systemic therapy.

- Types of systemic therapy include chemotherapy, immunotherapy, and targeted therapy. Systemic therapy might be used alone or with other therapies.

- Radiation therapy (RT) uses high-energy radiation from photons, electrons, or protons, and other sources to kill cancer cells and shrink tumors.

- A clinical trial is a type of research that studies a treatment to see how safe it is and how well it works.

Questions to ask

- Which treatment(s) do you recommend and why?

- What can I expect from treatment?

- How will you treat side effects? What should I look for?

- Are there resources to help pay for treatment or other care I may need?

- What clinical trial options are available?

4
Supportive care

37 What is supportive care?

37 Side effects

41 Late effects

41 Survivorship

41 Key points

41 Questions to ask

4 Supportive care » What is supportive care? » Side effects

Supportive care helps manage the symptoms of DLBCL and the side effects of treatment. This chapter discusses possible side effects.

What is supportive care?

Supportive care helps improve your quality of life during and after cancer treatment. The goal is to prevent or manage side effects and symptoms, like pain and cancer-related fatigue. It also addresses the mental, social, and spiritual concerns faced by those with cancer.

Supportive care is available to everyone with cancer and their families, not just those at the end of life. Palliative care is another name for supportive care.

Supportive care can also help with:

- Making treatment decisions
- Coordinating your care
- Paying for care
- Planning for advanced care and end of life

Side effects

All cancer treatments can cause unwanted health issues called side effects. Side effects depend on many factors. These factors include the drug type and dose, length of treatment, and the person. Some side effects may be unpleasant. Others may be harmful to one's health. Treatment can cause several side effects. Some are very serious. Tell your care team about any new or worsening symptoms.

You will be monitored throughout treatment for side effects or other unwanted (adverse) reactions. All systemic therapies may cause severe, life-threatening, or fatal reactions. Some potential side effects are described next. They are not listed in order of importance. Some side effects are very rare.

Blood clots

Cancer and cancer treatment can cause blood clots to form. This can block blood flow and oxygen in the body. Blood clots are often formed in the lower legs and can break loose and travel to other parts of the body causing breathing problems, strokes, or other problems.

Cytokine release syndrome

Cytokine release syndrome (CRS) is a condition that may occur after treatment with some types of immunotherapy, such as monoclonal antibodies and CAR T cells. It is caused by a large, rapid release of inflammatory proteins called cytokines from immune cells affected by the immunotherapy. Signs and symptoms of CRS include fever, muscle aches, nausea, headache, rash, fast heartbeat, low blood pressure, and trouble breathing.

Diarrhea

Diarrhea is frequent and watery bowel movements. Your care team will tell you how to manage diarrhea. It is important to drink lots of fluids.

4 Supportive care » Side effects

Distress

Depression, anxiety, and sleeping problems are common and are a normal part of cancer diagnosis. Talk to your care team with those whom you feel most comfortable about how you may be feeling. There are services, people, and medicine that can help you and your loved ones and caregivers. Support and counseling services are available.

Fatigue

Fatigue is extreme tiredness and inability to function due to lack of energy. Fatigue may be caused by cancer or it may be a side effect of treatment. Let your care team know how you are feeling and if fatigue is getting in the way of you doing the things you enjoy. Eating a balanced diet and physical activity can help. You might be referred to a nutritionist or dietitian to help with fatigue.

Hair loss

Chemotherapy may cause hair loss (alopecia) all over your body—not just on your scalp. Some chemotherapy drugs are more likely than others to cause hair loss. Dosage might also affect the amount of hair loss. Most of the time, hair loss from chemotherapy is temporary. Hair often regrows 3 to 6 months after treatment ends. Your hair may be a different shade or texture at first.

Hypersensitivity, allergy, and anaphylaxis

Certain treatments can cause an unwanted reaction. Hypersensitivity is an exaggerated response by the immune system to a drug or other substance. This can include hives, skin welts, and trouble breathing. An allergy is an immune reaction to a substance that normally is harmless or would not cause an immune response in most people. An allergic response may cause harmful symptoms such as itching or inflammation (swelling). Anaphylaxis or anaphylactic shock is a severe and possible life-threatening allergic reaction.

> **All cancer treatments can cause unwanted health issues called side effects. It is important to tell your care team about all of your side effects so they can be managed.**

Infections

Infections occur more frequently and are more severe in those with a weakened immune system. Drug treatment for lymphoma can weaken the body's natural defense against infections. If not treated early, infections can be fatal.

Neutropenia, a low number of white blood cells, can lead to frequent or severe infections. When someone with neutropenia also develops a fever, it is called febrile neutropenia (FN). With FN, your risk of infection may be higher than normal. This is because a low number of white blood cells leads to a reduced ability to fight infections. FN is a side effect of some types of systemic therapy. **It is important to notify your care team immediately of any fevers while you may be neutropenic.**

Loss of appetite

Sometimes side effects from cancer or its treatment, and the stress of having cancer might cause you to feel not hungry or sick to your stomach (nauseated). You might have a sore mouth or difficulty swallowing. Healthy eating is important during treatment, even when you don't have an appetite or get pleasure from eating. It includes eating a balanced diet, eating the right amount of food, and drinking enough fluids. A registered dietitian who is an expert in nutrition and food can help. Speak to your care team if you have trouble eating or maintaining weight.

Low blood cell counts

Some cancer treatments can cause low blood cell counts.

- **Anemia** is a condition where your body does not have enough healthy red blood cells, resulting in less oxygen being carried to your body tissues. You might tire easily or feel short of breath if you are anemic.
- **Neutropenia** is a decrease in neutrophils, the most common type of white blood cell. This puts you at risk for severe infection.
- **Thrombocytopenia** is a condition where there are not enough platelets found in the blood. This puts you at risk for bleeding.

Lymphedema

Lymphedema is a condition in which lymph fluid builds up in tissues and causes swelling. It may be caused when part of the lymph system is damaged or blocked, such as during surgery to remove lymph nodes, or by radiation therapy. Cancers that block lymph vessels can also cause lymphedema. Swelling usually develops slowly over time. It may develop during treatment, or it may start years after treatment. If you have lymphedema, you may be referred to an expert in lymphedema management. The swelling may be reduced by exercise, massage, compression devices, and other means.

Nausea and vomiting

Nausea and vomiting are common side effects of treatment. You will be given medicine to prevent nausea and vomiting.

Neurocognitive or neuropsychological effects

Some treatments can damage the nervous system (neurotoxicity) causing problems with concentration and memory. Survivors are at risk for neurotoxicity and might be recommended for neuropsychological testing. Neuropsychology looks at how the health of your brain affects your thinking and behavior. Neuropsychological testing can identify your limits and doctors can create a plan to help with these limits.

Neuropathy and neurotoxicity

Some treatments can damage the nervous system (neurotoxicity) causing neuropathy and problems with concentration, memory, and thinking. Neuropathy is a nerve problem that causes pain, numbness, tingling, swelling, or muscle weakness in different parts of the body. It usually begins in the hands or feet and gets worse with additional cycles of treatment. Let your care team know if you are experiencing these symptoms so they can determine if

4 Supportive care » Side effects

any changes to the dose of your treatment is needed. Most of the time, neuropathy improves gradually and may eventually go away after treatment.

Organ issues

Treatment might cause your kidneys, liver, and heart to not work as well as they should.

Pain

Tell your care team about any pain or discomfort. You might meet with a palliative care specialist or with a pain specialist to manage pain.

Palliative care

Palliative care is appropriate for anyone, regardless of age, cancer stage, or the need for other therapies. It focuses on physical, emotional, social, and spiritual needs that affect quality of life.

Quality of life

Cancer and its treatment can affect your overall well-being or quality of life (QOL). For more information on quality of life, see *NCCN Guidelines for Patients: Palliative Care* at NCCN.org/patientguidelines and on the NCCN Patient Guides for Cancer app.

Therapy-related toxicity

Many of the drug therapies used to treat diffuse large B-cell lymphomas can be harmful to the body. You will be closely monitored for therapy-related toxicity.

Tumor lysis syndrome

Cancer treatment causes cell death. In tumor lysis syndrome (TLS), waste released by dead cancer cells builds up in the body causing kidney damage and severe blood electrolyte disturbances. Changes in creatinine, lactic acid, uric acid, phosphorus (Phos), potassium (K), and calcium (Ca) levels can be a sign of TLS. TLS is rare.

Supportive care resources

More information on supportive care is available at NCCN.org/patientguidelines and on the NCCN Patient Guides for Cancer app.

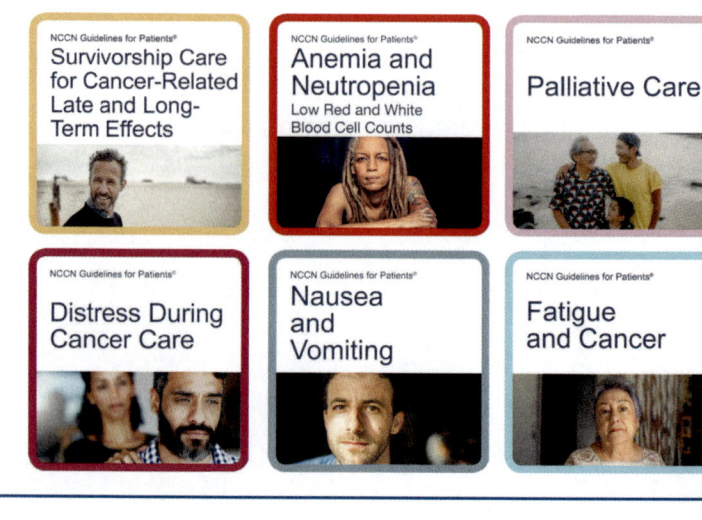

Weight gain

Weight gain is one side effect of high-dose steroids. This can be uncomfortable and cause distress. It is important to maintain muscle mass. Find a physical activity you enjoy. Ask your care team what can be done to help manage weight gain.

Late effects

Late effects are side effects that occur months or years after a disease is diagnosed or after treatment has ended. Late effects may be caused by cancer or cancer treatment. They may include physical, mental, and social health issues, and second cancers. The sooner late effects are treated the better. Ask the care team about what late effects could occur. This will help you know what to look for.

Survivorship

A person is a cancer survivor from the time of diagnosis until the end of life. After treatment, your health will be monitored for side effects of treatment and the return of cancer. This is part of a survivorship care plan. It is important to keep any follow-up doctor visits and imaging test appointments. Find out who will coordinate your follow-up care.

Key points

- Supportive care is health care that relieves symptoms caused by cancer or its treatment and improves quality of life.
- All cancer treatments can cause unwanted health issues called side effects. Side effects depend on many factors. These factors include the drug type and dose, length of treatment, and the person.
- Some side effects are very rare. Ask your care team what to expect.
- Tell your care team about any new or worsening symptoms.

Questions to ask

- What are the side effects of this treatment?
- How are these side effects treated?
- What should I do if I notice changes in my condition?
- What should I do on weekends and other non-office hours?
- Will my care team be able to communicate with the emergency department or urgent care team?

5
Stages 1, 2, 3, and 4

43 Staging

44 Stages 1 and 2 non-bulky (limited)

45 Stages 1 and 2 bulky (limited)

46 Stages 3 and 4

47 Follow-up testing

48 Key points

48 Questions to ask

5 Stages 1, 2, 3, and 4 » Staging

Treatment for DLBCL is based on cancer stage and is often a combination of chemoimmunotherapy and radiation therapy. Together, you and your care team will choose a treatment plan that is best for you.

Staging

A PET and/or CT scan will be done to stage diffuse large B-cell lymphoma (DLBCL). In addition, treatment decisions will be based on histology and results of biomarker and genetic tests. Histology is the overall appearance and the size, shape, and type of your cells.

In general, stages for DLBCL are as follows:

> **Stage 1 (limited)** – Disease found in 1 lymph node or a group of nearby lymph nodes.

> **Stage 2 (limited)** – Disease found in 2 or more lymph node groups on the same side of the diaphragm.

> **Stage 2 bulky** – Bulky disease means there are areas of lymphoma that measure 7.5 centimeters (cm) or larger. Bulky disease can be limited or advanced.

> **Stage 3 (advanced)** – Disease found in lymph nodes above and below the diaphragm, or disease found in nodes above the diaphragm and in the spleen.

> **Stage 4 (advanced)** – Disease has spread outside of the lymphatic system to other parts of the body.

Lymph node regions

Lymph node regions based on the Ann Arbor Staging System

Adapted from: Lymph_node_regions.jpg: https://commons.wikimedia.org/wiki/File:Lymph_node_regions.svg

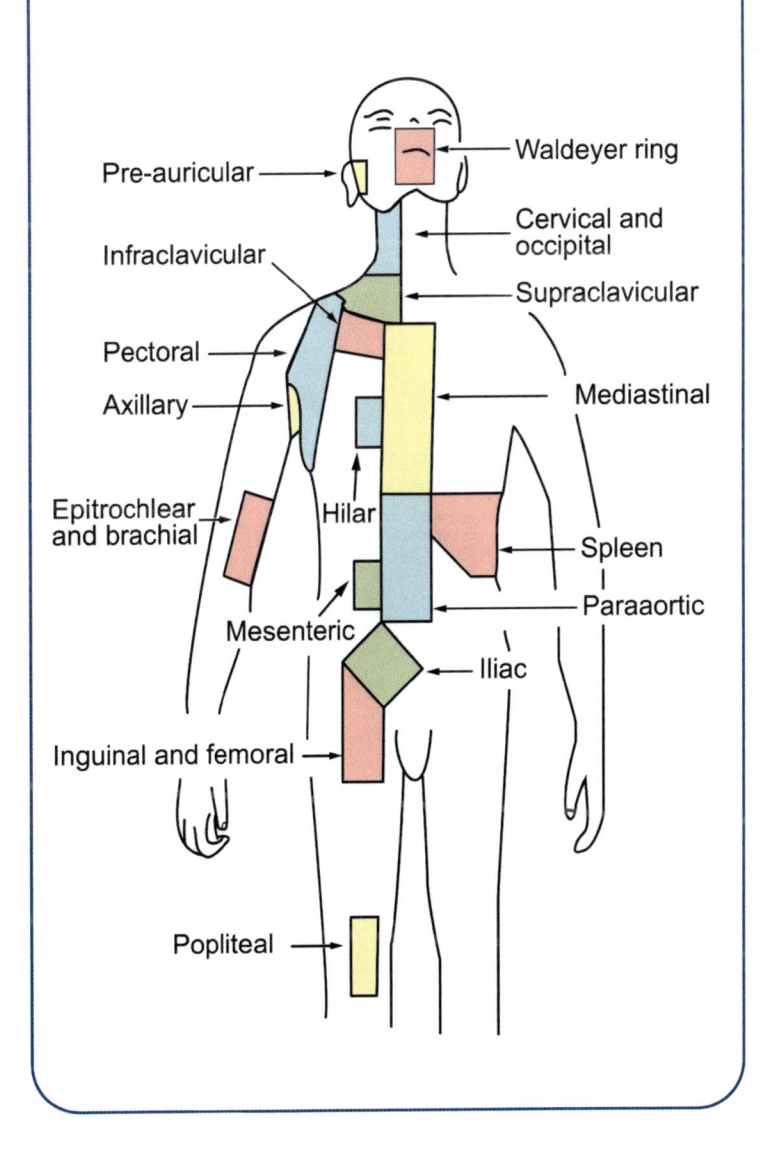

Stages 1 and 2 non-bulky (limited)

Initial treatment for non-bulky stage 1 or 2 limited disease is 3 cycles of RCHOP. This is called first-line chemoimmunotherapy. Your cancer will be restaged using PET/CT after 3 cycles of RCHOP and again after the last cycle.

› If a complete response, you will have 1 more cycle of RCHOP for a total of 4 cycles or involved-site radiation therapy (ISRT). Then, you will enter surveillance and be monitored for relapse.

› If a partial response, you will have 1 to 3 more cycles of RCHOP for a total of 4 to 6 cycles or ISRT if PET scan was positive for disease after 3 cycles of RCHOP.

› If disease has progressed, a repeat biopsy will be done, and you will be treated for refractory disease found in *Chapter 6: Relapsed and refractory disease.*

Stage 2 DLBCL

In stage 2 DLBCL, cancer is found in 2 or more lymph node groups on the same side of the diaphragm.

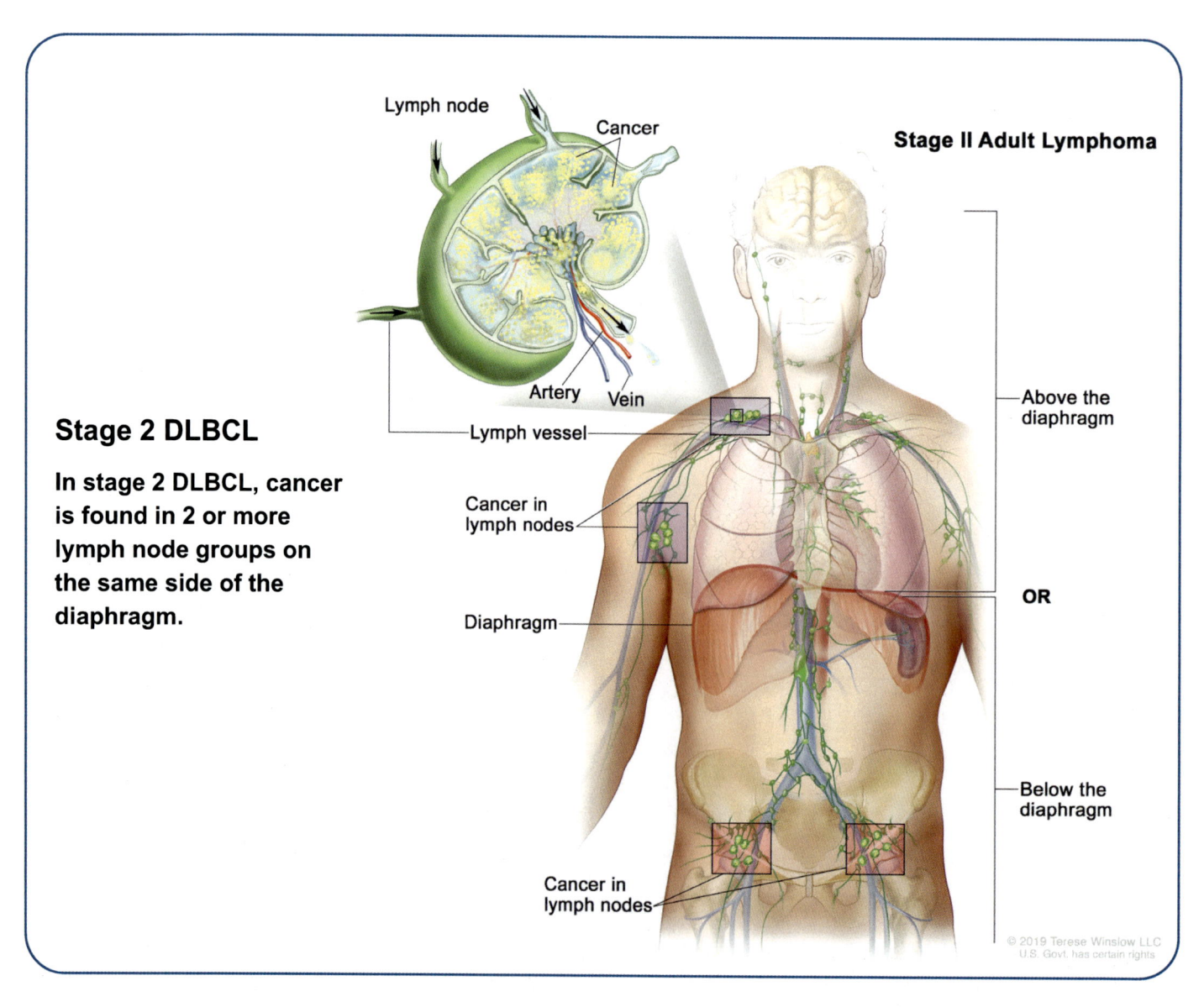

5 Stages 1, 2, 3, and 4 » Stages 1 and 2 bulky (limited)

Stages 1 and 2 bulky (limited)

Bulky disease in DLBCL refers to cancer that is 7.5 cm or larger. Treatment for stage 1 or 2 limited, bulky disease is 6 total cycles of RCHOP. This is called first-line chemoimmunotherapy. A type of radiation called involved-site radiation therapy (ISRT) might be added.

Your cancer will be restaged using PET/CT after 3 to 4 cycles of RCHOP and again after the last (6th) cycle.

> If a complete response, you will complete the planned course of treatment. If in remission, also called a complete response, then you will enter surveillance and be monitored for relapse.

> If a partial response, you will complete the planned course of treatment.

> If no treatment response or disease has progressed, a repeat biopsy will be done and you will be treated for refractory disease found in *Chapter 6: Relapsed and refractory disease.*

International Prognostic Index

The International Prognostic Index (IPI) is a scoring system to predict prognosis in those with lymphoma. A prognosis is the likely course your disease will take. IPI is based on age, performance status (PS), the stage of the cancer, lactate dehydrogenase (LDH) results, and if cancer is found in more than one area besides the lymph nodes.

5 Stages 1, 2, 3, and 4 » Stages 3 and 4

Stages 3 and 4

For stages 3 and 4, chemoimmunotherapy such as RCHOP and Pola-R-CHP are the recommended and preferred options. Other chemotherapy regimens such as DA-EPOCH-R might be used for those with certain types of DLBCL and in persons with HIV. A CT or PET scan might be done after 2 to 4 cycles to restage your cancer. For all first-line therapy options, **see Guide 4**.

> If a complete or partial response, you will finish the remaining cycles of treatment for a total of 6 cycles. Then, you will enter surveillance and be monitored for relapse.

> If no treatment response or disease has progressed, a repeat biopsy will be done and you will be treated for refractory disease found in *Chapter 6: Relapsed and refractory disease.*

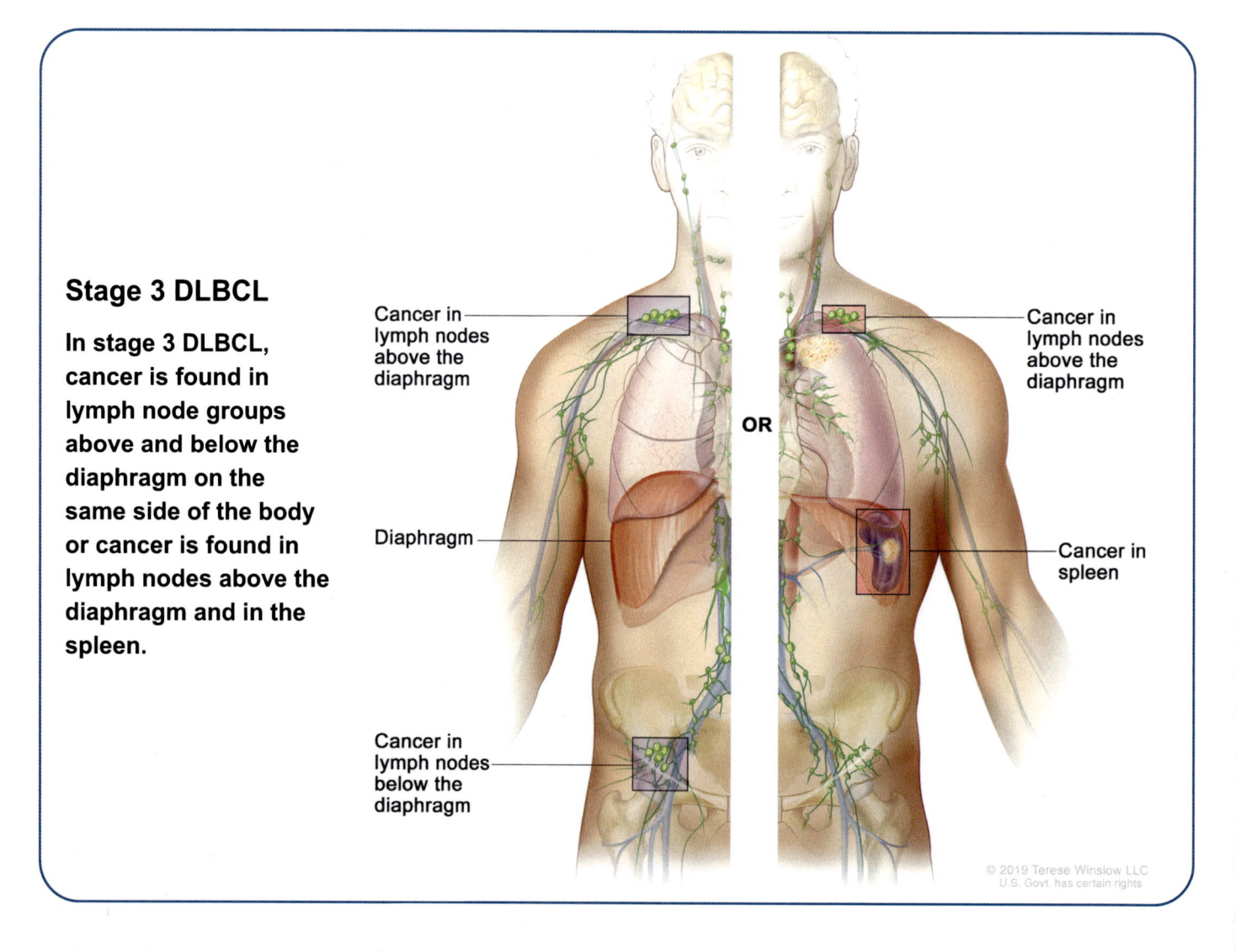

Stage 3 DLBCL

In stage 3 DLBCL, cancer is found in lymph node groups above and below the diaphragm on the same side of the body or cancer is found in lymph nodes above the diaphragm and in the spleen.

Cancer in lymph nodes above the diaphragm

Diaphragm

Cancer in lymph nodes below the diaphragm

OR

Cancer in lymph nodes above the diaphragm

Cancer in spleen

© 2019 Terese Winslow LLC
U.S. Govt. has certain rights

NCCN Guidelines for Patients®
Diffuse Large B-Cell Lymphomas, 2025

5 Stages 1, 2, 3, and 4 » Follow-up testing

Follow-up testing

After completing all cycles of treatment, a PET/CT scan will be done. Radiation therapy might be considered based on the initial stage of disease or response to treatment. Surveillance is a period of testing that begins after remission to monitor for the return of cancer. It includes physical exam, health history, and blood tests every 3 to 6 months for 5 years.

After 5 years, testing will be done once a year or as needed.

Surveillance imaging may be considered for monitoring those without symptoms (asymptomatic). This may include a chest/abdomen/pelvis CT no more than every 6 months for 2 years. After 2 years, imaging testing will be done as needed. Discuss with your care team if surveillance imaging is right for you.

Guide 4
First-line therapy options

Preferred options	• Cyclophosphamide, doxorubicin, vincristine, and prednisone with rituximab (RCHOP) • Polatuzumab vedotin-piiq, rituximab, cyclophosphamide, doxorubicin and prednisone (Pola-R-CHP)
Other recommended	• Dose-adjusted etoposide, prednisone, vincristine, cyclophosphamide, and doxorubicin with rituximab (DA-EPOCH-R)
For those with heart issues	• Dose-adjusted etoposide, prednisone, vincristine, cyclophosphamide, doxorubicin, and rituximab (DA-EPOCH-R) • Rituximab, cyclophosphamide, liposomal doxorubicin, vincristine, and prednisone (RCDOP) • Rituximab, cyclophosphamide, etoposide, vincristine, and prednisone (RCEOP) • Rituximab, gemcitabine, cyclophosphamide, vincristine, and prednisone (RGCVP) • Rituximab, cyclophosphamide, etoposide, prednisone, and procarbazine (RCEPP)
For those who are frail or are over 80 years of age with other health issues	• Rituximab, cyclophosphamide, liposomal doxorubicin, vincristine, and prednisone (RCDOP) • Rituximab with mini-CHOP (R-mini-CHOP) • Rituximab, gemcitabine, cyclophosphamide, vincristine, and prednisone (RGCVP) • Rituximab, cyclophosphamide, etoposide, prednisone, and procarbazine (RCEPP)

*An FDA-approved biosimilar might be used in place of rituximab.

Key points

- RCHOP is chemoimmunotherapy that consists of rituximab, cyclophosphamide, doxorubicin, vincristine, and prednisone.

- Treatment for non-bulky stage 1 or 2 disease is 4 to 6 cycles of RCHOP.

- Bulky disease in DLBCL refers to cancer that is 7.5 cm or larger. Treatment for bulky stage 1 or 2 disease is 6 cycles of RCHOP.

- For stages 3 and 4, chemoimmunotherapy such as RCHOP and Pola-R-CHP are the recommended and preferred options. Other chemoimmunotherapy regimens might be used.

- A type of radiation called ISRT might be added to treatment. Involved-site radiation therapy (ISRT) treats cancer found in a small region or one area of your body.

- Surveillance is a period of testing that begins after remission to monitor for relapse or the return of cancer.

Questions to ask

- How does my risk group affect the treatment options?

- Does the order of treatments matter?

- Which treatment do you recommend and why?

- Are there any other doctors I need to meet to finalize my treatment plan?

- What side effects can I expect from this treatment?

6
Relapsed and refractory disease

50 Relapse – Under 12 months

52 Relapse – Over 12 months

53 Refractory disease

54 2 or more relapses

54 Follow-up testing

55 Key points

55 Questions to ask

6 Relapsed and refractory disease » Relapse – Under 12 months

Cancer that returns is called relapse. The goal of treatment is to achieve remission again. When DLBCL progresses during treatment, it is called refractory. Together, you and your care team will choose a treatment plan that is best for you.

Relapse – Under 12 months

Treatment options for relapsed disease are based on the time since your last treatment was completed. If cancer returned and it has been less than 12 months since treatment ended, then treatment will be based on if CAR T-cell therapy is planned.

CAR T-cell therapy is planned

CD19-targeting CAR T-cell therapy is an option for relapse that has occurred less than 12 months since treatment ended. CD19-targeting CAR T-cell therapy options include axicabtagene ciloleucel and lisocabtagene maraleucel. While waiting for CAR T-cell therapy, bridging therapy will be given as needed. **See Guide 5.**

Guide 5
CAR T-cell bridging therapy options

Dexamethasone and cytarabine (DHA) with carboplatin, cisplatin, or oxaliplatin
Gemcitabine, dexamethasone, and cisplatin (GDP) or gemcitabine, dexamethasone, and carboplatin
Gemcitabine and oxaliplatin (GemOx)
Ifosfamide, carboplatin, and etoposide (ICE)
Polatuzumab vedotin-piiq with or without rituximab with or without bendamustine
Involved-site radiation therapy (ISRT)
*Rituximab might be added to the therapies listed. An FDA-approved biosimilar might be used for rituximab.

6 Relapsed and refractory disease » Relapse – Under 12 months

CAR T-cell therapy not planned

If CAR T-cell therapy is not planned, then options include as follows:

> Clinical trial
> Second-line therapy, **see Guide 6**
> Palliative involved-site radiation therapy (ISRT)
> Best supportive care to improve quality of life

After a complete response, you will have follow-up testing.

After a partial response, no response, or disease progression, see treatment for 2 or more relapses on page 54.

Guide 6
Second-line therapy options

Preferred options	• Epcoritamab-bysp with GemOx • Glofitamab-gxbm with GemOx • Polatuzumab vedotin-piiq with or without bendamustine with or without rituximab • Polatuzumab vedotin-piiq and mosunetuzumab-axgb • Tafasitamab-cxix and lenalidomide
Other recommended	• Cyclophosphamide, etoposide, vincristine, and prednisone (CEOP). • Dexamethasone and cytarabine (DHA) with carboplatin, cisplatin, or oxaliplatin • Etoposide, methylprednisolone, cytarabine, and cisplatin (ESHAP) • Gemcitabine, dexamethasone, and cisplatin (GDP) • Gemcitabine and oxaliplatin (GemOx) • Ifosfamide, carboplatin, and etoposide (ICE) • Mesna, ifosfamide, mitoxantrone, and etoposide (MINE) • Rituximab might be added to therapies in this list.
Used in some cases	• Brentuximab vedotin • Ibrutinib • Lenalidomide with or without rituximab

*An FDA-approved biosimilar might be used in place of rituximab.

NCCN Guidelines for Patients®
Diffuse Large B-Cell Lymphomas, 2025

6 Relapsed and refractory disease » Relapse – Over 12 months

Relapse – Over 12 months

For cancer that returned after more than 12 months since treatment ended, treatment options are described next.

HCT is planned

If autologous (self) hematopoietic cell transplant (HCT) is planned, then second-line therapy will be given. **See Guide 7.**

After a complete response, next options include:

- Autologous HCT. ISRT might be added.
- Clinical trial
- In some cases, an allogeneic (donor) HCT
- Involved-site radiation therapy (ISRT) might be added. ISRT treats lymph nodes where cancer was originally found or cancer located in a small region or one area of your body.

After a partial response, next options include:

- CAR T-cell therapy. Bridging therapy might be given. **See Guide 5.**
- Autologous HCT. ISRT might be added.
- Clinical trial
- In some cases, an allogeneic (donor) HCT. ISRT might be added.

If no response or disease progression, then see treatment for 2 or more relapses on page 54.

Guide 7
Second-line therapy options: HCT planned

Preferred options	• Dexamethasone and cytarabine (DHA) with carboplatin, cisplatin, or oxaliplatin • Gemcitabine, dexamethasone, and cisplatin (GDP) or gemcitabine, dexamethasone, and carboplatin • Ifosfamide, carboplatin, and etoposide (ICE)
Other recommended	• Etoposide, methylprednisolone, cytarabine, and cisplatin (ESHAP) • Gemcitabine and oxaliplatin (GemOx) • Mesna, ifosfamide, mitoxantrone, and etoposide (MINE)

*Rituximab might be added to any of the therapies listed above. An FDA-approved biosimilar might be used in place of rituximab.

6 Relapsed and refractory disease » Refractory disease

HCT not planned

If you are not receiving a hematopoietic cell transplant (HCT), then options include:

- Clinical trial
- Second-line therapy, **see Guide 8**
- Palliative ISRT
- Best supportive care

After a complete response, you will have follow-up testing.

After a partial response, no response, or disease progression, see treatment for 2 or more relapses on page 54.

Refractory disease

Refractory disease might be treated with CAR T-cell therapy. While waiting for CAR T-cell therapy, bridging therapy will be given as needed. For bridging therapy, **see Guide 5.**

Other options include:

- Clinical trial
- Second-line therapy, **see Guide 6**
- Palliative ISRT
- Best supportive care
- RT with or without chemoimmunotherapy followed by autologous HCT may be an option in some people with localized disease.

Guide 8
Second-line therapy options: HCT not planned

Preferred options	• CD19-targeting CAR T-cell therapy (lisocabtagene maraleucel) • Epcoritamab-bysp with GemOx • Glofitamab-gxbm with GemOx • Polatuzumab vedotin-piiq with or without bendamustine with or without rituximab • Polatuzumab vedotin-piiq and mosunetuzumab-axgb • Tafasitamab-cxix and lenalidomide
Other recommended	• Cyclophosphamide, etoposide, vincristine, and prednisone (CEOP). Rituximab might be added. • Gemcitabine, dexamethasone, and cisplatin (GDP). Rituximab might be added. • Gemcitabine and oxaliplatin (GemOx). Rituximab might be added. • Rituximab alone
Used in some cases	• Brentuximab vedotin • Ibrutinib • Lenalidomide with or without rituximab

*An FDA-approved biosimilar might be used in place of rituximab.

6 Relapsed and refractory disease » 2 or more relapses » Follow-up testing

After a complete response, you will have follow-up testing.

After a partial response, no response, or disease progression, see treatment for 2 or more relapses next.

2 or more relapses

For a partial response, second or third relapse, or disease progression, then the treatment options include:

> Third-line therapy, **see Guide 9**
> A systemic therapy not used before
> Clinical trial

> Palliative ISRT
> Best supportive care

If a complete or partial response to treatment, an allogeneic (donor) HCT with or without ISRT might be an option in some cases.

Follow-up testing

After completing treatment, you will have the following tests to monitor for relapse:

> A physical exam, health history, and blood tests every 3 to 6 months for 5 years. After 5 years, these tests will be done once a year or as needed.

Guide 9 **Third-line and next-line therapy options**	
Preferred options	CD19-targeting CAR T-cell therapy (preferred if not previously given) • Axicabtagene ciloleucel • Lisocabtagene maraleucel • Tisagenlecleucel
	Bispecific antibody therapy (only after at least two lines of systemic therapy; including those with disease progression after HCT or CAR T-cell therapy) • Epcoritamab-bysp • Glofitamab-gxbm
Other recommended	• Brentuximab vedotin and lenalidomide with rituximab (for CD30+ disease) • Loncastuximab tesirine-lpyl • Selinexor (including those with disease progression after HCT or CAR T-cell therapy)

*An FDA-approved biosimilar might be used in place of rituximab.

NCCN Guidelines for Patients®
Diffuse Large B-Cell Lymphomas, 2025

6 Relapsed and refractory disease » Key points » Questions to ask

- Surveillance imaging may be considered for those without symptoms (asymptomatic). This may include a chest/abdomen/pelvis CT no more than every 6 months for 2 years. After 2 years, imaging testing will be done as needed. Discuss with your care team if surveillance imaging is right for you

It is important to keep any follow-up doctor visits and imaging test appointments. Seek good routine medical care, including regular doctor visits for preventive care and cancer screening.

Key points

- Cancer that returns is called relapse. Treatment options for relapsed disease are based on the time since treatment was completed. The goal of treatment is to achieve remission again.

- If cancer returned and it has been less than 12 months since treatment ended, then treatment will be based on if CAR T-cell therapy is planned.

- If cancer returned after more than 12 months since treatment ended, then treatment will be based on if a hematopoietic cell transplant (HCT) is planned.

- When DLBCL progresses during treatment, it is called refractory. Refractory disease might be treated with CAR T-cell therapy. Other treatment options are available.

- After completing treatment, you will be monitored for the return of cancer. Keep all follow-up doctor visits and imaging test appointments.

Questions to ask

- Which treatment do you recommend and why?

- Why are some treatment options preferred over others?

- Does this treatment offer a cure? If not, how well can treatment stop the cancer from growing?

- Does the order of treatments matter?

- Is a hematopoietic cell transplant (HCT), CAR T-cell therapy, or a clinical trial an option for me?

7
ALK-positive large B-cell lymphomas

57 Overview

57 Treatment

58 Key points

58 Questions to ask

7 ALK-positive large B-cell lymphomas » Overview » Treatment

ALK-positive large B-cell lymphoma (ALK+ LBCL) is caused by a mutation in the *ALK* gene. ALK+ LBCL is usually treated with radiation therapy and chemotherapy. Together, you and your care team will choose a treatment plan that is best for you.

Overview

ALK-positive large B-cell lymphoma (ALK+ LBCL) is caused by a mutation in the anaplastic lymphoma kinase (*ALK*) gene. *ALK* tells your body how to make proteins that help cells talk to each other. ALK+ LBCL expresses the ALK protein but lacks CD20 (CD20-). The *ALK* mutation makes this lymphoma difficult to treat.

ALK+ LBCL is not associated with immune deficiency. Epstein-Barr virus (EBV) and Kaposi sarcoma-associated herpesvirus (HHV8) are negative. A gene fusion called *CLTC::ALK* is common in ALK+ LBCL. It is written as t(2;17)(p23;q23).

Most with ALK+ LBCL have advanced disease with cancer found inside and outside the lymph nodes. Cancer found inside the lymph nodes is called nodal disease. Cancer found outside the lymph nodes is called extranodal. ALK+ LBCL is more commonly seen in those around 40 years of age, and sex assigned as male at birth.

Treatment

Currently, there is no standard of care or agreement on treatment. ALK+ LBCL is usually treated with chemotherapy. Involved-site radiation therapy (ISRT) is preferred when treating localized disease. A clinical trial is recommended if available and it is what you want. Since this cancer is often CD20-, rituximab is not given.

First-line treatment options include:

- Clinical trial (recommended)
- ISRT (preferred for localized disease)
- DA-EPOCH
- CHOEP
- CHOP
- Mini-CHOP
- HyperCVAD
- CODOX-M/IVAC

Treatment options for relapse or refractory disease include:

- Clinical trial (recommended)
- A platinum-based chemotherapy followed by an autologous (self) hematopoietic cell transplant (HCT). Platinum-based chemotherapy includes carboplatin, cisplatin, or oxaliplatin.
- Second-generation ALK inhibitors such as alectinib and lorlatinib followed by an allogeneic (donor) HCT.

7 ALK-positive large B-cell lymphomas » Key points » Questions to ask

Key points

- ALK-positive large B-cell lymphoma (ALK+ LBCL) is caused by a mutation in the *ALK* gene.

- A gene fusion called *CLTC::ALK* is common in ALK+ LBCL. It is written as t(2;17)(p23;q23).

- Most with ALK+ LBCL have advanced disease with cancer found inside and outside the lymph nodes.

- ALK+ LBCL is usually treated with radiation therapy and chemotherapy.

- A clinical trial is recommended if available and it is what you want.

- Treatment for relapse or refractory disease might be a hematopoietic cell transplant (HCT).

Questions to ask

- Which treatment do you recommend and why?

- Does this treatment offer a cure? If not, how well can treatment stop the cancer from growing?

- What side effects can I expect from this treatment?

- Does the order of treatments matter?

- Is a hematopoietic cell transplant (HCT) or a clinical trial an option for me?

8
Primary mediastinal large B-cell lymphomas

60 Overview

61 Treatment

62 Follow-up testing

62 Relapse or refractory disease

63 Key points

63 Questions to ask

8 Primary mediastinal large B-cell lymphomas » Overview

Primary mediastinal large B-cell lymphoma (PMBL) develops in the area behind the breastbone called the mediastinum. Treatment is chemoimmunotherapy. Together, you and your care team will choose a treatment plan that is best for you.

Overview

In primary mediastinal large B-cell lymphoma (PMBL), a tumor forms most often behind the breastbone (sternum). This can cause a cough, shortness of breath, or swelling of the head and neck, due to the tumor pressing on the windpipe and the large veins above the heart. Enlarged lymph nodes in this area can also be found. PMBL can spread to organs and tissues such as the lungs, pericardium (sac around the heart), liver, gastrointestinal (GI) tract, ovaries, adrenal glands, and central nervous system (CNS).

PMBL is more commonly seen in those 30 to 40 years of age, assigned female at birth.

Abnormal chromosomes are common in PMBL. An expert hematopathologist review is essential to confirm the diagnosis of PMBL.

Mediastinum

Mediastinal lymphomas are growths found in the area of the chest that separates the lungs called the mediastinum. In primary mediastinal large B-cell lymphoma (PMBL), a tumor often forms behind the breastbone.

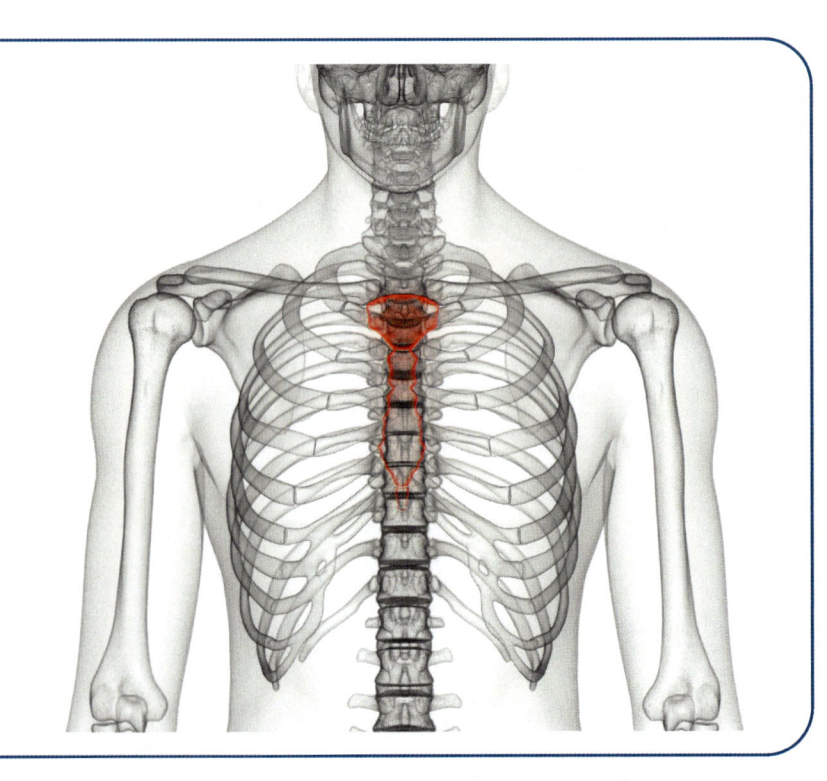

Treatment

Currently, the most used treatment options are:

- 6 cycles of DA-EPOCH-R (dose-adjusted etoposide, prednisone, vincristine, cyclophosphamide, and doxorubicin with rituximab).
- 4 to 6 cycles of RCHOP-14 (rituximab, cyclophosphamide, doxorubicin, vincristine, and prednisone).
- 6 cycles of RCHOP-21 (rituximab, cyclophosphamide, doxorubicin, vincristine, and prednisone).

A PET/CT scan will be given after treatment to restage your cancer. Some of the tumor tends to remain after treatment and a PET/CT will help find any residual masses. A biopsy might be done.

After a complete response

- After DA-EPOCH-R, you will enter observation.
- After 6 cycles of RCHOP-14, you will enter observation.
- After 6 cycles of RCHOP-21, you might have involved-site radiation therapy (ISRT) to treat cancer found in a small region or one area of your body.
- After 4 cycles of RCHOP-14, you may have 3 cycles of ifosfamide, carboplatin, and etoposide (ICE). Rituximab might be added (RICE).

It is very important to continue to take your medicine as prescribed and not miss or skip any doses.

After a partial response or cancer progresses

If there is a partial response or cancer progresses, biopsy may be repeated. If cancer remains, then ISRT might be given or one of the following:

- Pembrolizumab
- Nivolumab with or without brentuximab vedotin
- Or treat as in *Chapter 6: Relapsed and refractory disease*

Follow-up testing

After a complete response (remission), you will be monitored for relapse with the following tests:

› A physical exam, health history, and blood tests every 3 to 6 months for 5 years. After 5 years, these tests will be done once a year or as needed.

› Surveillance imaging may be considered for monitoring those without symptoms (asymptomatic). This may include a chest/abdomen/pelvis CT no more than every 6 months for 2 years. After 2 years, imaging testing will be done as needed. Discuss with your care team if surveillance imaging is right for you.

Relapse or refractory disease

Cancer that returns is called relapse. When cancer progresses despite treatment, it is called refractory.

Treatment options include:

› Treatment options vary by type of DLBCL, whether disease was refractory to initial therapy, and timing of relapse. Treatment options may include different chemoimmunotherapy regimens from initial therapy, CAR-T therapy, or HCT.

› Or treat as in *Chapter 6: Relapsed and refractory disease*.

"My diagnosis was sudden and unexpected. I am a non-smoker and runner and had just completed a half marathon before diagnosis. My only symptom was a persistent cough. My tumor was causing fluid to back up in my heart and lungs."

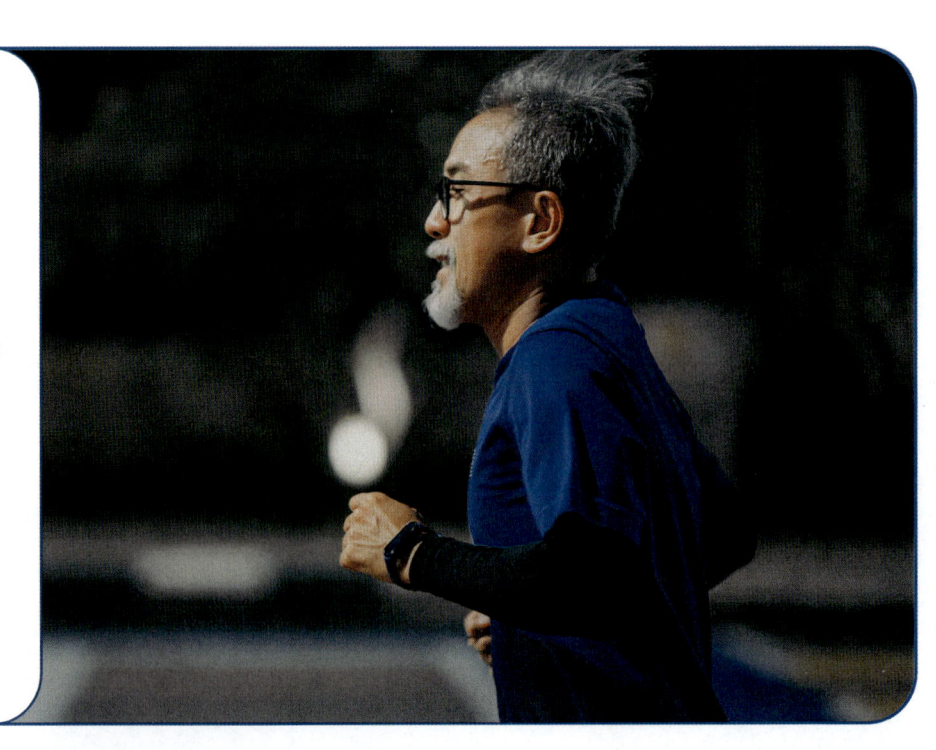

8 Primary mediastinal large B-cell lymphomas » Key points » Questions to ask

Key points

- In primary mediastinal large B-cell lymphoma (PMBL), a tumor forms most often behind the breastbone (sternum).
- Treatment is chemoimmunotherapy.
- After a complete response (remission), you will be monitored for relapse.
- Immunotherapy such as pembrolizumab or nivolumab with or without brentuximab vedotin (an antibody drug conjugate), CAR-T therapy, or an HCT might be used to treat cancer that has progressed, relapsed, or is refractory.

Questions to ask

- Which treatment do you recommend and why?
- Does this treatment offer a cure? If not, how well can treatment stop the cancer from growing?
- What side effects can I expect from this treatment?
- Does the order of treatments matter?
- What is the likelihood this cancer will return?

9
High-grade B-cell lymphomas

65 Overview

65 HGBL with *MYC* and *BCL2*

65 HGBL with *MYC* and *BCL6*

66 HGBL, not otherwise specified

66 Relapse and refractory disease

67 Key points

67 Questions to ask

9 High-grade B-cell lymphomas » Overview » *MYC* and *BCL2* » *MYC* and *BCL6*

High-grade B-cell lymphomas (HGBLs) are very aggressive, fast-dividing tumors. This chapter will provide information on HGBL with gene rearrangements and HGBL, not otherwise specified (HGBL, NOS). Together, you and your care team will choose a treatment plan that is best for you.

Overview

High-grade B-cell lymphomas (HGBLs) have mutations, gene rearrangements such as *MYC*, or other high-risk features that make treatment a challenge. Those with HGBL often have an elevated lactate dehydrogenase (LDH), bone marrow and central nervous system (CNS) involvement, and a high International Prognostic Index (IPI) score. Since cancer is often found in the bone marrow and central nervous system, a lumbar puncture might be done. In addition, intrathecal (IT) chemotherapy might be given at the time of a lumbar puncture to prevent CNS disease.

Currently, there is no standard of care or agreement on treatment for HGBLs. Treatment is usually chemoimmunotherapy. Radiation therapy might be given. A clinical trial is recommended, if available and it is what you want.

HGBL with *MYC* and *BCL2*

Those with HGBL with gene rearrangements of *MYC* and *BCL2* are treated as follows:

- Clinical trial (recommended)
- ISRT (preferred for localized disease)
- DA-EPOCH-R
- RCHOP
- R-mini-CHOP
- R-HyperCVAD
- R-CODOX-M/R-IVAC

HGBL with *MYC* and *BCL6*

HGBL with gene rearrangements of *MYC* and *BCL6* is often treated with DA-EPOCH-R or other systemic therapies used for DLBCL. See Guide 4 on page 47.

9 High-grade B-cell lymphomas » HGBL, not otherwise specified

HGBL, not otherwise specified

HGBL, not otherwise specified (HGBL-NOS) includes tumors that aren't well defined or don't fall into another HGBL category.

Treatment options include:

- Clinical trial (recommended)
- ISRT for localized disease
- DA-EPOCH-R
- Pola-R-CHP
- RCHOP
- R-mini-CHOP
- R-HyperCVAD
- R-CODOX-M/R-IVAC

Relapse and refractory disease

For relapse and refractory disease treatment options, see *Chapter 6: Relapsed and refractory disease.*

Chemoimmunotherapy regimens

- **DA-EPOCH-R** is dose-adjusted etoposide, prednisone, vincristine, cyclophosphamide, doxorubicin, and rituximab.

- **Pola-R-CHP** is polatuzumab vedotin-piiq, rituximab, cyclophosphamide, doxorubicin, and prednisone.

- **RCHOP** is rituximab, cyclophosphamide, doxorubicin, vincristine, and prednisone.

- **R-HyperCVAD** is rituximab, cyclophosphamide, vincristine, doxorubicin, and dexamethasone alternating with high-dose methotrexate and cytarabine.

- **R-CODOX-M/R-IVAC** is rituximab, cyclophosphamide, vincristine, doxorubicin, and methotrexate alternating with rituximab, ifosfamide, etoposide, and cytarabine.

9 High-grade B-cell lymphomas » Key points » Questions to ask

Key points

- High-grade B-cell lymphomas (HGBLs) are aggressive, fast-dividing tumors.
- Those with HGBL have elevated LDH, bone marrow and CNS involvement, and a high IPI score.
- A clinical trial is recommended for those with HGBL. Treatment options may include radiation therapy for localized disease and chemoimmunotherapy.
- HGBL, not otherwise specified (HGBL-NOS) includes tumors that aren't well defined or don't fall into another HGBL category.

Questions to ask

- Which treatment do you recommend and why?
- Does this treatment offer a cure? If not, how well can treatment stop the cancer from growing?
- What side effects can I expect from this treatment?
- Does the order of treatments matter?
- Is a hematopoietic cell transplant (HCT) or a clinical trial an option for me?

10
Mediastinal gray zone lymphomas

69 Overview

70 Treatment

71 Key points

71 Questions to ask

10 Mediastinal gray zone lymphomas » Overview

Mediastinal gray zone lymphoma (MGZL) has overlapping features of primary mediastinal B-cell lymphoma (PMBL) and Hodgkin lymphoma (HL). Treatment is usually chemotherapy. Together, you and your care team will choose a treatment plan that is best for you.

> **Mediastinal gray zone lymphoma (MGZL) is different than primary mediastinal large B-cell lymphoma (PMBL). Those with gray zone lymphomas are best managed in cancer centers with experience in treating this type of lymphoma.**

Overview

Gray zone lymphomas have overlapping features of non-Hodgkin primary mediastinal B-cell lymphoma (PMBL) and Hodgkin lymphoma (HL). This means that the cells are large but can vary in size and might look similar to Hodgkin cells (Reed-Sternberg cells). Reed-Sternberg cells are large, abnormal lymphocytes that may contain more than one nucleus.

There are 2 main types of gray zone lymphomas:

> Mediastinal gray zone lymphoma (MGZL)
> Non-mediastinal gray zone lymphomas

Mediastinal gray zone lymphomas

Mediastinal lymphomas are growths found behind the breastbone (sternum) in the part of the chest that separates the lungs and holds the heart. Mediastinal gray zone lymphoma (MGZL) is different than primary mediastinal large B-cell lymphoma (PMBL). They are treated differently. Primary mediastinal lymphomas are discussed in Chapter 8.

MGZLs are more commonly seen in those between 20 to 40 years of age, assigned male at birth. They are characterized by the presence of a large mediastinal mass. Lymph nodes above the collar bone (supraclavicular) may be involved.

An expert hematopathologist review is essential to confirm the diagnosis of mediastinal gray zone lymphoma.

Non-mediastinal gray zone lymphomas

Non-mediastinal gray zone lymphomas occur in older persons, have a higher rate of bone marrow involvement, include disease outside the lymph nodes (extranodal disease), and have more advanced-stage disease than mediastinal gray zone lymphomas. However, those with cancer found outside the mediastinum (extra-mediastinal disease) should be diagnosed as having DLBCL, not otherwise specified (DLBCL-NOS), see page 42.

10 Mediastinal gray zone lymphomas » Treatment

Treatment

Since MGZL has features of both classical Hodgkin lymphoma (CHL) and non-Hodgkin PMBL, treatment is a challenge. Currently, there is no standard of care or agreement on treatment. MGZL is usually treated with chemotherapy. If the tumor cells are CD20+, rituximab might be added to chemotherapy. This is called chemoimmunotherapy. Involved-site radiation therapy (ISRT) may be added in those with localized disease.

For possible systemic therapy options, **see Guide 9.**

Guide 9
Systemic therapy options: Mediastinal gray zone lymphomas

Preferred options	• Cyclophosphamide, doxorubicin, vincristine, and prednisone with rituximab (RCHOP) • Polatuzumab vedotin-piiq, rituximab, cyclophosphamide, doxorubicin and prednisone (Pola-R-CHP)
Other recommended	• Dose-adjusted etoposide, prednisone, vincristine, cyclophosphamide, and doxorubicin with rituximab (DA-EPOCH-R)
For those with heart issues	• Dose-adjusted etoposide, prednisone, vincristine, cyclophosphamide, doxorubicin, and rituximab (DA-EPOCH-R) • Rituximab, cyclophosphamide, liposomal doxorubicin, vincristine, and prednisone (RCDOP) • Rituximab, cyclophosphamide, etoposide, vincristine, and prednisone (RCEOP) • Rituximab, gemcitabine, cyclophosphamide, vincristine, and prednisone (RGCVP) • Rituximab, cyclophosphamide, etoposide, prednisone, and procarbazine (RCEPP)
For those who are frail or are over 80 years of age with other health issues	• Rituximab, cyclophosphamide, liposomal doxorubicin, vincristine, and prednisone (RCDOP) • Rituximab with mini-CHOP (R-mini-CHOP) • Rituximab, gemcitabine, cyclophosphamide, vincristine, and prednisone (RGCVP) • Rituximab, cyclophosphamide, etoposide, prednisone, and procarbazine (RCEPP)

*An FDA-approved biosimilar might be used in place of rituximab.

Key points

- Gray zone lymphomas have overlapping features of primary mediastinal B-cell lymphoma (PMBL) and Hodgkin lymphoma (HL).

- There are 2 main types of gray zone lymphomas: mediastinal gray zone lymphomas and non-mediastinal gray zone lymphomas.

- Mediastinal lymphomas are growths found behind the breastbone (sternum) in the part of the chest that separates the lungs and holds the heart.

- An expert hematopathologist review is essential to confirm the diagnosis of MGZL.

- MGZL is usually treated with chemotherapy. Rituximab might be added to chemotherapy if the tumor cells are CD20+. Involved-site radiation therapy (ISRT) may be added in those with localized disease.

Questions to ask

- What can I expect from treatment and what are the risks?

- Does this treatment offer a cure?

- What side effects should I look for and when should I contact my care team?

- How can I prepare for the possibility of relapse?

- Will the treatment I choose today affect my choices if cancer relapses or is refractory?

11
Primary cutaneous DLBCL, leg type

73 Overview

74 Treatment

75 Solitary or regional disease

75 Generalized skin-only disease

75 Extracutaneous disease

76 Follow-up testing

76 Relapse and refractory disease

76 Key points

76 Questions to ask

11 Primary cutaneous DLBCL, leg type » Overview

In primary cutaneous diffuse large B-cell lymphoma (PC-DLBCL), leg type, abnormal B-cell lymphocytes cause skin lesions. Although the skin is involved, the skin cells themselves are not cancerous. Despite its name, PC-DLBCL, leg type can be found anywhere on the body. Treatment options are based on many factors. Together, you and your care team will choose a treatment plan that is best for you.

Overview

Primary cutaneous diffuse large B-cell lymphoma (PC-DLBCL), leg type consists of large, transformed B cells that typically appear as red or bluish-red tumors on the skin. Despite its name, the disease can involve the torso, arms, legs, buttocks, or anywhere on the body. PC-DLBCL, leg type can also spread to areas other than the skin. An expert hematopathologist review is essential to confirm the diagnosis of primary cutaneous DLBCL, leg type. A skin biopsy is done to distinguish between PC-DLBCL, leg type from other types of primary cutaneous lymphomas (lymphomas of the skin).

More information on other types of primary cutaneous lymphomas can be found in the *NCCN Guidelines for Patients: Cutaneous B-Cell Lymphomas* and *NCCN Guidelines for Patients: Cutaneous T-Cell Lymphomas*, available at NCCN.org/patientguidelines and on the NCCN Patient Guides for Cancer app.

"Drug treatment for DLBCL was intense and strong. And, I had unusual side effects. I told my care team right away when I noticed a side effect. This really helped. They were very good at treating it!"

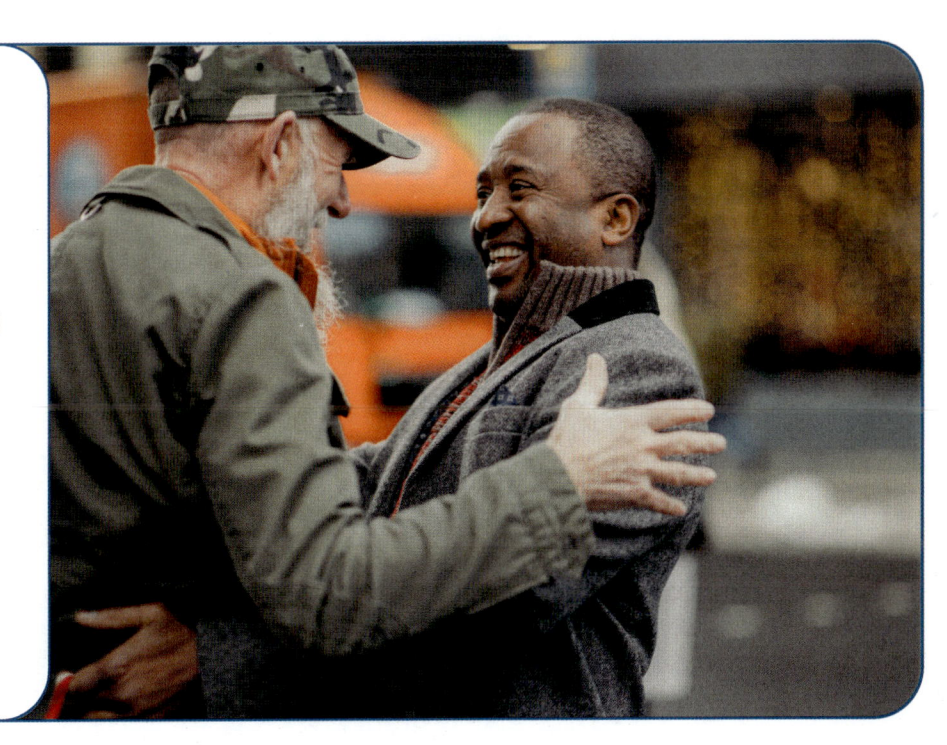

11 Primary cutaneous DLBCL, leg type » Treatment

Treatment

Treatment is based on the number of skin lesions and their location. This is called staging. Skin lesions/tumors (T) will be measured by their depth, height, size, and region of the body. Lesions are often measured in centimeters (cm). Body regions are based on regional lymph node drainage patterns. Body regions include head/neck, chest, upper arm, lower arm and hand, abdomen and genitals, upper leg, lower leg and feet, upper back, and lower back and buttocks.

Disease may be solitary, regional, generalized skin only, or outside the skin (extracutaneous). At the end of treatment, imaging tests are needed to assess response.

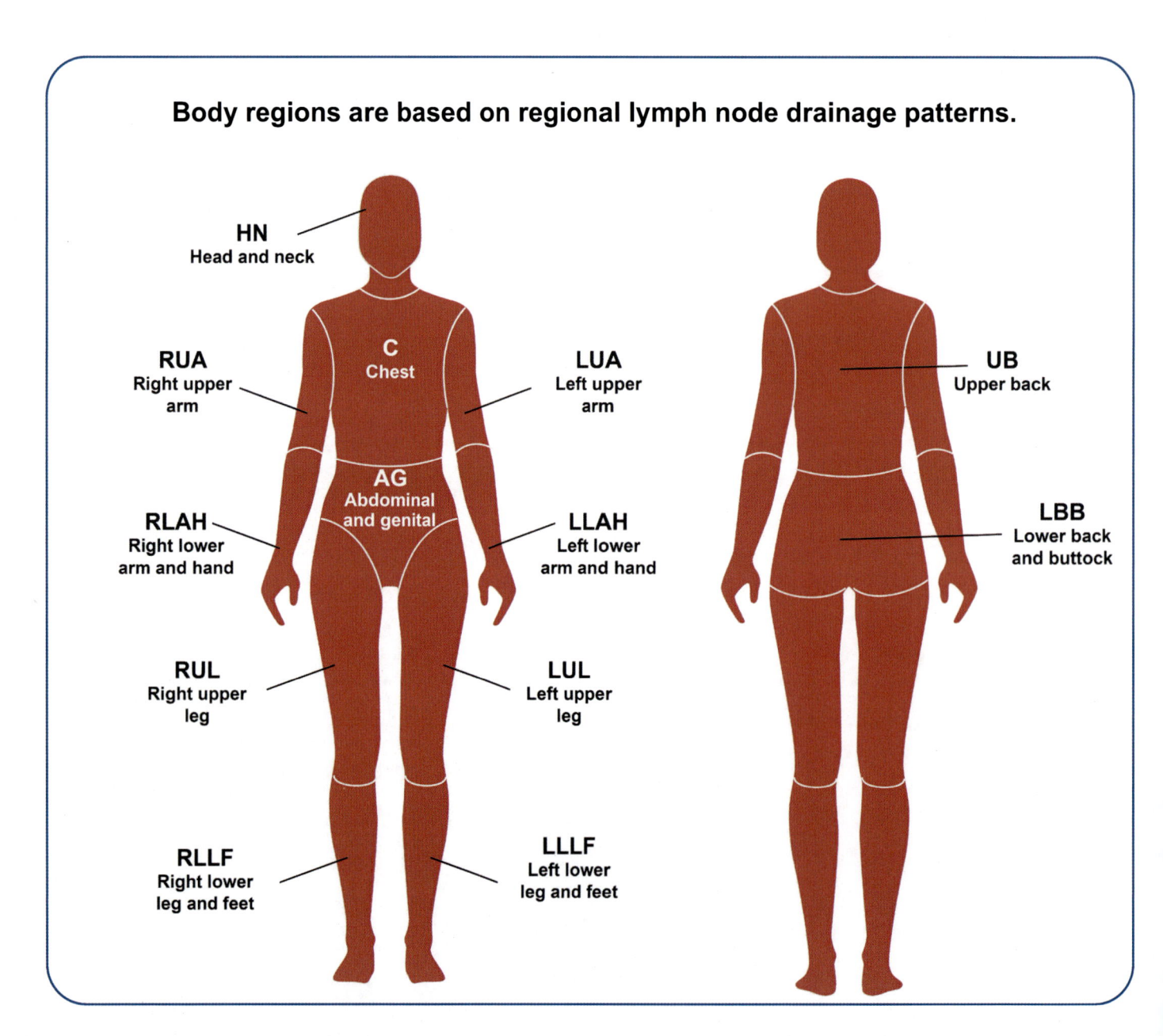

Body regions are based on regional lymph node drainage patterns.

- **HN** Head and neck
- **C** Chest
- **RUA** Right upper arm
- **LUA** Left upper arm
- **AG** Abdominal and genital
- **RLAH** Right lower arm and hand
- **LLAH** Left lower arm and hand
- **RUL** Right upper leg
- **LUL** Left upper leg
- **RLLF** Right lower leg and feet
- **LLLF** Left lower leg and feet
- **UB** Upper back
- **LBB** Lower back and buttock

NCCN Guidelines for Patients®
Diffuse Large B-Cell Lymphomas, 2025

11 Primary cutaneous DLBCL, leg type » Solitary or regional » Skin-only » Extracutaneous

Solitary or regional disease

A solitary lesion is one lesion (T1). Regional lesions can be multiple lesions limited to one body region or two adjoining regions (T2). Disease area will be measured.

Options include:

- RCHOP (rituximab, cyclophosphamide, doxorubicin, vincristine, and prednisone) with local involved-site radiation therapy (ISRT)
- Local ISRT
- Clinical trial

After a complete response (CR), you will have follow-up testing to monitor for relapse.

For a relapse, if not given before, you might be treated with RCHOP or local radiation therapy (ISRT). Other treatment options are based on if relapse occurred less than 12 months or more than 12 months since your initial treatment ended. For more information, see *Chapter 6: Relapsed and refractory disease*.

Generalized skin-only disease

Generalized skin-only disease covers a larger area of the body than regional disease. There are multiple lesions that involve 2 or more body regions (T3) not next to one another. Disease is not found in lymph nodes, blood, or other organs. Treatment works inside the body to target the skin lesions. ISRT might be used to target a specific area of skin.

First treatment

First-line therapy is the first treatment given. Skin-only disease is initially treated with RCHOP. RCHOP is rituximab, cyclophosphamide, doxorubicin, vincristine, and prednisone. ISRT might be added to treat the skin lesions. A clinical trial is also an option.

After a complete response, you will have imaging tests and be monitored for relapse with follow-up testing.

For a relapse, if not given before, you might be treated with RCHOP or local radiation therapy (ISRT). Other treatment options are based on if relapse occurred less than 12 months or more than 12 months since your initial treatment ended. For more information, see *Chapter 6: Relapsed and refractory disease*.

Next treatment or relapse

If there was no response, a partial response, or a relapse, then treatment will be:

- A different chemoimmunotherapy
- Palliative ISRT

Extracutaneous disease

Extracutaneous disease is found outside the skin. This is cancer that might be found in the lymph nodes, blood, or organs. Treatment will be based on the stage of diffuse large B-cell lymphoma (DLBCL) found in *Chapter 5: Stages 1, 2, 3, and 4*.

Follow-up testing

After a complete response (CR), you will be monitored for relapse with the following tests:

> A physical exam, health history, and blood tests every 3 to 6 months for 5 years. After 5 years, these tests will be done once a year or as needed.

> Surveillance imaging may be considered for monitoring those without symptoms (asymptomatic). This may include a chest/abdomen/pelvis CT no more than every 6 months for 2 years. After 2 years, imaging testing will be done as needed. Discuss with your care team if surveillance imaging is right for you.

Relapse and refractory disease

Treatment options are based on if relapse occurred less than 12 months or more than 12 months since your initial treatment ended. For more information, see *Chapter 6: Relapsed and refractory disease*.

Key points

> Primary cutaneous diffuse large B-cell lymphoma (PC-DLBCL), leg type consists of large, transformed B cells that typically appear as red or bluish-red tumors on the skin. It is not skin cancer.

> Despite its name, PC-DLBCL, leg type can be found anywhere on the body. Treatment is based on the number of skin lesions and their location. This is called staging.

> Disease may be solitary, regional, generalized skin only, or outside the skin (extracutaneous).

> A solitary lesion is one lesion (T1).

> Regional lesions can be multiple lesions limited to one body region or two adjoining regions (T2).

> Generalized skin-only disease covers a larger area of the body than regional disease. There are multiple lesions that involve 2 or more body regions (T3) not next to one another.

> Extracutaneous disease is disease that might be found in the lymph nodes, blood, or organs.

Questions to ask

> What can I expect from treatment and what are the risks?

> How can I find a dermatologist that specializes in PC-DLBCL?

> What side effects should I look for and when should I contact my care team?

> How can I prepare for the possibility of relapse?

> Will the treatment I choose today affect my choices if cancer relapses or is refractory?

12
Other resources

78 What else to know

78 What else to do

78 Where to get help

79 Questions to ask about resources and support

12 Other resources » What else to know » Where to get help

Want to learn more? Here's how you can get additional help.

What else to know

This book is an important tool for improving cancer care. It plainly explains expert recommendations and suggests questions to ask your care team. But, it's not the only resource that you have.

You're welcome to receive as much information and help as you need. Many people are interested in learning more about:

- The details of treatment
- Being a part of a care team
- Getting financial help
- Finding an oncologist who is an expert in DLBCL
- Coping with side effects

What else to do

Your health care center can help you with next steps. They often have on-site resources to help meet your needs and find answers to your questions. Health care centers can also inform you of resources in your community.

In addition to help from your providers, the resources listed in the next section provide support for many people like yourself. Look through the list and visit the provided websites to learn more about these organizations

Where to get help

AnCan Foundation
Ancan.org

Blood & Marrow Transplant Information Network (BMT InfoNet)
BMTInfoNet.org

CancerCare
Cancercare.org

Cancer Hope Network
cancerhopenetwork.org

HealthTree Foundation
Healthtree.org

Imerman Angels
Imermanangels.org

Lymphoma Research Foundation
lymphoma.org

MedlinePlus
medlineplus.gov

National Bone Marrow Transplant Link (nbmtLINK)
nbmtLINK.org

National Cancer Institute (NCI)
cancer.gov/types/lymphoma

National Coalition for Cancer Survivorship
canceradvocacy.org

12 Other resources » Questions to ask about resources and support

NMDP
nmdp.org

The Leukemia & Lymphoma Society (LLS)
LLS.org/PatientSupport

Triage Cancer
triagecancer.org

Questions to ask about resources and support

- Who can I talk to about help with housing, food, and other basic needs?
- What help is available for transportation, childcare, and home care?
- What other services are available to me and my caregivers?
- How can I connect with others and build a support system?
- Who can I talk to if I don't feel safe at home, at work, or in my neighborhood?

Let us know what you think!

Please take a moment to complete an online survey about the NCCN Guidelines for Patients.
NCCN.org/patients/response

Words to know

allogeneic hematopoietic cell transplant (allogeneic HCT)
A cancer treatment that replaces a person's bone marrow and immune system with donor cells to fight the lymphoma.

autologous hematopoietic cell transplant (autologous HCT)
A cancer treatment that destroys your bone marrow then rebuilds it with your healthy stem cells. Also called high-dose therapy with autologous stem cell rescue (HDT/ASCR). The high-dose therapy is used to eradicate the disease and stem cell rescue is needed because of the toxic effects of the treatment.

best supportive care
Treatment to improve quality of life and relieve discomfort.

biomarker testing
A lab test of any molecule in your body that can be measured to assess your health. Also called molecular testing.

biopsy
A procedure that removes fluid or tissue samples to be tested for a disease.

biosimilar
A drug that is almost an identical drug made by another company. It has been approved by the U.S. Food and Drug Administration (FDA) and must be used in the exact same way and at the same dose as the other drug.

bone marrow
The sponge-like tissue in the center of most bones.

bone marrow aspiration
A procedure that removes a liquid bone marrow sample to test for a disease.

bone marrow biopsy
A procedure that removes bone and solid bone marrow samples to test for a disease.

chemotherapy
Cancer drugs that stop the cell life cycle so that cells don't increase in number.

chromosome
The structures within cells that contain coded instructions for cell behavior.

clinical trial
A type of research that assesses health tests or treatments.

complete response (CR)
No signs of lymphoma are found. Also called complete remission.

computed tomography (CT)
A test that uses x-rays from many angles to make a picture of the insides of the body.

contrast
A substance put into your body to make clearer pictures during imaging tests.

deoxyribonucleic acid (DNA)
A chain of chemicals in cells that contains coded instructions for making and controlling cells.

flow cytometry
A lab test of substances on the surface of cells to identify the type of cells present.

Words to know

fluorescence in situ hybridization (FISH)
A lab test that uses special dyes to look for abnormal chromosomes and genes.

gene
A set of coded instructions in cells for making new cells and controlling how cells behave.

hematopathologist
A doctor who specializes in the study of blood diseases and cancers using a microscope.

hematopoietic cell transplant (HCT)
A cancer treatment that replaces a person's bone marrow and immune system with donor cells to fight the lymphoma.

high-grade B-cell lymphoma (HGBL)
A type of lymphoma that grows and spreads quickly and has severe symptoms.

histology
The study of tissues and cells under a microscope.

human leukocyte antigen (HLA)
A cell protein by which your body knows its own cells from foreign cells.

imaging test
A test that makes pictures (images) of the insides of the body.

immune system
The body's natural defense against infection and disease.

immunohistochemistry (IHC)
A lab test of cancer cells to find specific cell traits involved in abnormal cell growth.

immunophenotyping
A lab test that detects the type of cells present based on the cells' surface proteins.

induction
The first treatment that is given to greatly reduce the amount of cancer.

in situ hybridization (ISH)
A lab test of the number of a gene.

involved-site radiation therapy (ISRT)
Uses radiation therapy to treat cancer located in a small region or one area of your body.

karyotype
Lab test that makes a map of chromosomes to find defects.

lactate dehydrogenase (LDH)
A protein in blood that helps to make energy in cells.

lymph
A clear fluid containing white blood cells.

lymph node
A small, bean-shaped disease-fighting structure.

lymphadenopathy
Lymph nodes that are abnormal in size or consistency.

lymphatic system
Germ-fighting network of tissues and organs that includes the bone marrow, spleen, thymus, lymph nodes, and lymphatic vessels. Part of the immune system.

lymphocyte
A type of white blood cell that is part of the immune system.

magnetic resonance imaging (MRI)
A test that uses radio waves and powerful magnets to make pictures of the insides of the body.

mediastinal gray zone lymphoma (MGZL)
A type lymphoma with overlapping features of Hodgkin lymphoma (HL) and primary mediastinal large B-cell lymphoma (PMBL) found in the mediastinum (the area behind the breastbone).

Words to know

monitoring
A period of testing for changes in cancer status.

mutation
An abnormal change in the instructions within cells for making and controlling cells.

partial response (PR)
Lymphoma is still present but has reduced in size.

pathologist
A doctor who's an expert in testing cells and tissue to find disease.

peripheral blood (PB)
Blood that circulates throughout the body.

platelet (PLT)
A type of blood cell that helps control bleeding. Also called thrombocyte.

polymerase chain reaction (PCR)
A lab process in which copies of a DNA part are made.

positron emission tomography (PET)
A test that uses radioactive material to see the shape and function of body parts.

primary mediastinal large B-cell lymphoma (PMBL)
A fast-growing type of lymphoma that develops from B cells in the mediastinum (the area behind the breastbone).

prognosis
The likely course a disease will take.

radiation therapy (RT)
A treatment that uses high-energy rays.

recovery
A period of time without treatment to allow blood cell counts to return to normal.

recurrence
The return of cancer after a cancer-free period.

red blood cell (RBC)
A type of blood cell that carries oxygen from the lungs to the rest of the body. Also called an erythrocyte.

refractory cancer
A cancer that does not improve with treatment.

relapse
The return or worsening of cancer after a period of improvement.

remission
Minor or no signs of disease.

side effect
An unhealthy or unpleasant physical or emotional response to treatment.

supportive care
Treatment for the symptoms or health conditions caused by cancer or cancer treatment. Also sometimes called palliative care or best supportive care.

translocation
A switching of parts between two chromosomes.

tumor lysis syndrome (TLS)
A rare condition caused when waste released by dead cells is not quickly cleared out of your body.

white blood cell (WBC)
A type of blood cell that helps fight infections in the body. Also called a leukocyte.

NCCN Contributors

This patient guide is based on the NCCN Clinical Practice Guidelines in Oncology (NCCN Guidelines®) for B-Cell Lymphomas, Version 2.2025. It was adapted, reviewed, and published with help from the following people:

Dorothy A. Shead, MS
*Senior Director
Patient Information Operations*

Tanya Fischer, MEd, MSLIS
Senior Medical Writer

Susan Kidney
Senior Graphic Design Specialist

The NCCN Clinical Practice Guidelines in Oncology (NCCN Guidelines®) for B-Cell Lymphomas, Version 2.2025 were developed by the following NCCN Panel Members:

Andrew D. Zelenetz, MD, PhD/Chair
Memorial Sloan Kettering Cancer Center

Leo I. Gordon, MD/Vice Chair
Robert H. Lurie Comprehensive Cancer Center of Northwestern University

Jeremy S. Abramson, MD, MMSc
Mass General Cancer Center

Ranjana H. Advani, MD
Stanford Cancer Institute

Babis Andreadis, MD, MSCE
UCSF Helen Diller Family Comprehensive Cancer Center

Nancy L. Bartlett, MD
Siteman Cancer Center at Barnes-Jewish Hospital and Washington University School of Medicine

L. Elizabeth Budde, MD, PhD
City of Hope National Medical Center

Paolo F. Caimi, MD
Case Comprehensive Cancer Center/ University Hospitals Seidman Cancer Center and Cleveland Clinic Taussig Cancer Institute

Julie E. Chang, MD
University of Wisconsin Carbone Cancer Center

Beth Christian, MD
The Ohio State University Comprehensive Cancer Center - James Cancer Hospital and Solove Research Institute

Sven DeVos, MD, PhD
UCLA Jonsson Comprehensive Cancer Center

Bhagirathbhai Dholaria, MD
Vanderbilt-Ingram Cancer Center

Luis E. Fayad, MD
The University of Texas MD Anderson Cancer Center

Thomas M. Habermann, MD
Mayo Clinic Comprehensive Cancer Center

Muhammad Saad Hamid, MD
St. Jude Children's Research Hospital/ The University of Tennessee Health Science Center

Francisco Hernandez-Ilizaliturri, MD
Roswell Park Comprehensive Cancer Center

Boyu Hu, MD
Huntsman Cancer Institute at the University of Utah

*****Yasmin Karimi, MD**
University of Michigan Rogel Cancer Center

Christopher R. Kelsey, MD
Duke Cancer Institute

Rebecca King, MD
Mayo Clinic Comprehensive Cancer Center

Justin Kline, MD
The UChicago Medicine Comprehensive Cancer Center

Susan Krivacic, MPAff
Consultant

*****Ann S. LaCasce, MD, MMSc**
Dana-Farber/Brigham and Women's Cancer Center

Daniel J. Landsburg, MD
Abramson Cancer Center at the University of Pennsylvania

Megan Lim, MD, PhD
Memorial Sloan Kettering Cancer Center

Marcus Messmer, MD
Fox Chase Cancer Center

Rachel Rabinovitch, MD
University of Colorado Cancer Center

Praveen Ramakrishnan, MD, MS
UT Southwestern Simmons Comprehensive Cancer Center

*****Erin Reid, MD**
UC San Diego Moores Cancer Center

Kenneth B. Roberts, MD
Yale Cancer Center/Smilow Cancer Hospital

Hayder Saeed, MD
Moffitt Cancer Center

Naoyuki G. Saito, MD, PhD
Indiana University Melvin and Bren Simon Comprehensive Cancer Center

Stephen D. Smith, MD
Fred Hutchinson Cancer Center

Lode J. Swinnen, MBChB, MD
Johns Hopkins Kimmel Cancer Center

Joseph Tuscano, MD
UC Davis Comprehensive Cancer Center

Julie M. Vose, MD, MBA
Fred & Pamela Buffett Cancer Center

NCCN

Mary Dwyer, MS
Senior Director, Guidelines Operations

Hema Sundar, PhD
Senior Manager, Global Clinical Content

* Reviewed this patient guide. For disclosures, visit NCCN.org/disclosures.

NCCN Guidelines for Patients®
Diffuse Large B-Cell Lymphomas, 2025

NCCN Cancer Centers

Abramson Cancer Center
at the University of Pennsylvania
Philadelphia, Pennsylvania
800.789.7366 • pennmedicine.org/cancer

Case Comprehensive Cancer Center/
University Hospitals Seidman Cancer Center and
Cleveland Clinic Taussig Cancer Institute
Cleveland, Ohio
UH Seidman Cancer Center
800.641.2422 • uhhospitals.org/services/cancer-services
CC Taussig Cancer Institute
866.223.8100 • my.clevelandclinic.org/departments/cancer
Case CCC
216.844.8797 • case.edu/cancer

City of Hope National Medical Center
Duarte, California
800.826.4673 • cityofhope.org

Dana-Farber/Brigham and Women's Cancer Center |
Mass General Cancer Center
Boston, Massachusetts
877.442.3324 • youhaveus.org
617.726.5130 • massgeneral.org/cancer-center

Duke Cancer Institute
Durham, North Carolina
888.275.3853 • dukecancerinstitute.org

Fox Chase Cancer Center
Philadelphia, Pennsylvania
888.369.2427 • foxchase.org

Fred & Pamela Buffett Cancer Center
Omaha, Nebraska
402.559.5600 • unmc.edu/cancercenter

Fred Hutchinson Cancer Center
Seattle, Washington
206.667.5000 • fredhutch.org

Huntsman Cancer Institute at the University of Utah
Salt Lake City, Utah
800.824.2073 • healthcare.utah.edu/huntsmancancerinstitute

Indiana University Melvin and Bren Simon
Comprehensive Cancer Center
Indianapolis, Indiana
888.600.4822 • www.cancer.iu.edu

Johns Hopkins Kimmel Cancer Center
Baltimore, Maryland
410.955.8964
www.hopkinskimmelcancercenter.org

Mayo Clinic Comprehensive Cancer Center
Phoenix/Scottsdale, Arizona
Jacksonville, Florida
Rochester, Minnesota
480.301.8000 • Arizona
904.953.0853 • Florida
507.538.3270 • Minnesota
mayoclinic.org/cancercenter

Memorial Sloan Kettering Cancer Center
New York, New York
800.525.2225 • mskcc.org

Moffitt Cancer Center
Tampa, Florida
888.663.3488 • moffitt.org

O'Neal Comprehensive Cancer Center at UAB
Birmingham, Alabama
800.822.0933 • uab.edu/onealcancercenter

Robert H. Lurie Comprehensive Cancer
Center of Northwestern University
Chicago, Illinois
866.587.4322 • cancer.northwestern.edu

Roswell Park Comprehensive Cancer Center
Buffalo, New York
877.275.7724 • roswellpark.org

Siteman Cancer Center at Barnes-Jewish Hospital
and Washington University School of Medicine
St. Louis, Missouri
800.600.3606 • siteman.wustl.edu

St. Jude Children's Research Hospital/
The University of Tennessee Health Science Center
Memphis, Tennessee
866.278.5833 • stjude.org
901.448.5500 • uthsc.edu

Stanford Cancer Institute
Stanford, California
877.668.7535 • cancer.stanford.edu

The Ohio State University Comprehensive Cancer Center -
James Cancer Hospital and Solove Research Institute
Columbus, Ohio
800.293.5066 • cancer.osu.edu

The UChicago Medicine Comprehensive Cancer Center
Chicago, Illinois
773.702.1000 • uchicagomedicine.org/cancer

The University of Texas MD Anderson Cancer Center
Houston, Texas
844.269.5922 • mdanderson.org

NCCN Cancer Centers

UC Davis Comprehensive Cancer Center
Sacramento, California
916.734.5959 • 800.770.9261
health.ucdavis.edu/cancer

UC San Diego Moores Cancer Center
La Jolla, California
858.822.6100 • cancer.ucsd.edu

UCLA Jonsson Comprehensive Cancer Center
Los Angeles, California
310.825.5268 • uclahealth.org/cancer

UCSF Helen Diller Family Comprehensive Cancer Center
San Francisco, California
800.689.8273 • cancer.ucsf.edu

University of Colorado Cancer Center
Aurora, Colorado
720.848.0300 • coloradocancercenter.org

University of Michigan Rogel Cancer Center
Ann Arbor, Michigan
800.865.1125 • rogelcancercenter.org

University of Wisconsin Carbone Cancer Center
Madison, Wisconsin
608.265.1700 • uwhealth.org/cancer

UT Southwestern Simmons Comprehensive Cancer Center
Dallas, Texas
214.648.3111 • utsouthwestern.edu/simmons

Vanderbilt-Ingram Cancer Center
Nashville, Tennessee
877.936.8422 • vicc.org

Yale Cancer Center/Smilow Cancer Hospital
New Haven, Connecticut
855.4.SMILOW • yalecancercenter.org

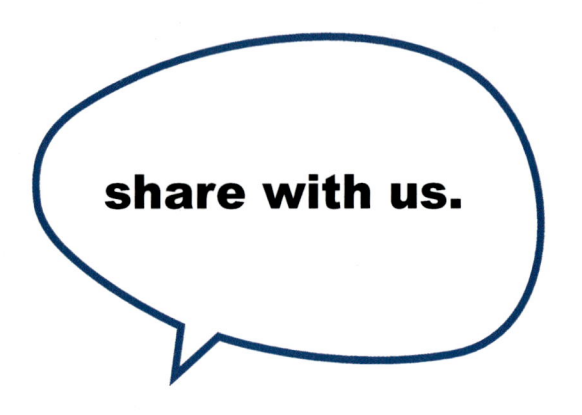

share with us.

Take our survey and help make the NCCN Guidelines for Patients better for everyone!

NCCN.org/patients/comments

Notes

Index

allogeneic hematopoietic cell transplant (HCT) 32

antibody drug conjugate (ADC) 30–31

antibody therapy 29–30

autologous hematopoietic cell transplant (HCT) 32

BCL2, BCL6, or *MYC* 19–20, 65

biomarker testing 18–21

biopsy 15–16

bispecific antibody therapy 30

bone marrow biopsy 16

CAR T-cell therapy 29

CD19-targeting CAR T-cell therapy 29

CD20-targeting therapy 30

chemoimmunotherapy 29

chemotherapy 28

clinical trials 33–34

computed tomography (CT) 21–22

DA-EPOCH-R 66

gene rearrangements 19–20

genetic cancer risk testing 21

genetic testing 18–21

heart tests 23

hematopoietic cell transplant (HCT) 32–33

human immunodeficiency virus (HIV) 14, 46

human leukocyte antigen (HLA) typing 14

immunophenotype 16–18

immunotherapy 29–30

induction 26

International Prognostic Index (IPI) 45

involved-site radiation therapy (ISRT) 32

large B-cell lymphoma (LBCL) subtypes 10

lumbar puncture (LP) 23

monoclonal antibody therapy (mAb) 29–30

mutations 18–19

performance status (PS) 13

Pola-R-CHP 29, 66

positron emission tomography (PET) 22–23

radiation therapy (RT) 31–32

RCHOP 29, 66

refractory 27

relapse 27

remission or complete response (CR) 27

side effects 37–41

surgery 33

surveillance or monitoring 27

survivorship 41

systemic therapy 28–31

targeted therapy 31

Made in the USA
Middletown, DE
20 September 2025